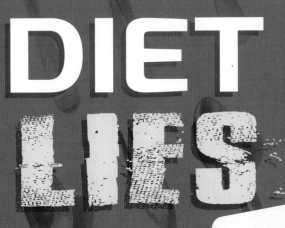

DIET LIES

AND

WEIGHT LOSS TRUTHS

A scientific guide to making sense out of dieting and exercise

Melody Schoenfeld, MA, CSCS, with **Susan Kleiner**, PhD, RD

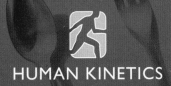

HUMAN KINETICS

Library of Congress Cataloging-in-Publication Data

Names: Schoenfeld, Melody, 1973- author. | Kleiner, Susan M., author.
Title: Diet lies and weight loss truths : a scientific guide to making
  sense out of dieting and exercise / Melody Schoenfeld with Susan
  Kleiner, RDN.
Description: Champaign, IL : Human Kinetics, [2021] | Includes
  bibliographical references and index.
Identifiers: LCCN 2020038089 (print) | LCCN 2020038090 (ebook) | ISBN
  9781718202412 (paperback) | ISBN 9781718202429 (epub) | ISBN
  9781718202436 (pdf)
Subjects: LCSH: Reducing diets. | Weight loss. | Exercise.
Classification: LCC RM222.2 .S336 2021 (print) | LCC RM222.2 (ebook) |
  DDC 613.2/5--dc23
LC record available at https://lccn.loc.gov/2020038089
LC ebook record available at https://lccn.loc.gov/2020038090

ISBN: 978-1-7182-0241-2 (print)

Senior Acquisitions Editor: Michelle Maloney; **Managing Editor:** Miranda K. Baur; **Copyeditor:** Michael Goldstein; **Indexer:** Rebecca McCorkle; **Permissions Manager:** Martha Gullo; **Senior Graphic Designer:** Joe Buck; **Cover Designer:** Keri Evans; **Cover Design Specialist:** Susan Rothermel Allen; **Photographs (interior):** Meredith M. Carlson unless otherwise noted; **Photo Asset Manager:** Laura Fitch; **Photo Production Manager:** Jason Allen; **Senior Art Manager:** Kelly Hendren; **Illustrations:** © Human Kinetics; **Printer:** Versa Press

Printed in the United States of America

10 9 8 7 6 5 4 3 2 1

The paper in this book is certified under a sustainable forestry program.

Human Kinetics

1607 N. Market Street
Champaign, IL 61820
USA

United States and International

Website: **US.HumanKinetics.com**
Email: info@hkusa.com
Phone: 1-800-747-4457

Canada

Website: **Canada.HumanKinetics.com**
Email: info@hkcanada.com

E8257

Tell us what you think!
Human Kinetics would love to hear what we
can do to improve the customer experience.
Use this QR code to take our brief survey.

DIET LIES

AND

WEIGHT LOSS TRUTHS

A scientific guide to making sense out of dieting and exercise

CONTENTS

Part II

Part III

PREFACE

by Melody Schoenfeld

I know what you're thinking.

"Oh, great. Another weight loss book."

And you'd be totally right for thinking that. The fact of the matter is, the weight loss industry has created a lot of millionaires (and continues to do so). All you have to do is come up with the next "Magical Ultimate Secret to Giving You That Body You've Always Wanted."

I make no such promises, because there is no such magic.

If you're looking for a meal plan, some restrictive diet scheme, or some magical ingredient that will change your life, this is not the book for you.

If you're looking for "The Ultimate One-Size-Fits-All Overnight Six Pack Abs Workout," this is not the book for you.

If you're confused by all the information out there, if you've been on a million diets without success, if you've been thinking about a specific diet and want to know more about it, or if you just like reading about diet science—well, this might very well be the book for you.

I am writing this book in order to clarify the current science on current diet trends. I explain what works, what may be problematic, and do a little myth busting on some of the lies that are told to sell you a specific plan. We are constantly bombarded with conflicting information, and, let's face it, it's confusing and headache inducing. Think of this book as me throwing my coat over the muddy pool of information for you to cross over and hopefully not get your shoes too dirty.

So, just for the time being, try to stop rolling your eyes at the thought of yet another weight loss book, and join me in an exploration of making lasting lifestyle changes. Hopefully, you won't ever have to read another weight loss book again.

INTRODUCTION

by Susan M. Kleiner, PhD, RD

Yep, it's true. All diets work . . . for somebody. Collectively, we're all dieting experts: going on a diet to go off it, just to try the next one. Finding a plan that you can stick with for the rest of your life is like discovering a pot of gold at the end of a rainbow. While the pot of gold may be a myth, finding your last diet is not. But you do need some help to separate the truths from the lies. This book will do that for you.

The world of diet and exercise is full of mythology, quackery, and fraud. It is very difficult to distinguish objective guidance from biased recommendations. While one would think that going to the original scientific literature should be the easiest way to identify unbiased authorship, today we have some published scientific authors who do not disclose their conflicts of interest and some scientific journals that do not require statements of possible conflicts of interest by authors. Even highly educated professionals can struggle to interpret the honesty of some publications. The truth is hard to find in books, magazines, documentaries, and websites that start with a kernel of truth and then omit entire bodies of evidence and twist words to prejudice their story and influence their audiences.

The diet industry has been built on evangelism underpinned by a system of unfounded beliefs and mysticism to keep sales churning, rather than scientific facts in which evidence carries the decisive edge. Consumers can be confounded by this misdirection for a while, but when it just doesn't work for them, they want real answers.

All is not lost! There is real science, with real evidence, and there are real answers. As with most things that are personal, you must determine which answer is right for you to achieve your goals. The only way you can figure that out is to have real information guiding the choices that you make for yourself.

Melody has done the detective work for you in *Diet Lies and Weight Loss Truths* in an absolutely clear and understandable way. You'll learn science without feeling like you need to become a scientist, and you'll understand diets without needing to become a dietitian. It's as if she's standing next to you in the gym or at a party and you asked her about the latest diet you want to try. You'll learn the high points and low points of each diet. You'll be able to decide whether it's the diet plan that will get you to your goals for the last and final time or the one that you cross off your list completely.

I strongly recommend that you start at the beginning of this book and not rush to the end, where you think you might find the ultimate answer. Finding a solution nearly always requires understanding the problem, evaluating the obstacles, and then planning the strategy to achieve success. Part I will offer information to help you understand the problem and obstacles in your path. What are the basic concepts of a successful weight loss plan? What difficulties might you encounter? How can you evaluate marketing strategies and hard selling techniques to sift through the hype to get to the facts? What's the lowdown on the 12 popular diet styles discussed in this book?

Part II will guide you through diet-planning strategies to create solutions that work for you, avoiding the lies and pitfalls of the dark side of the diet world. You'll even get to see sample menus of nutrition strategies that, according to research data, support both health and weight loss. These are the kinds of plans you can follow forever.

Part III is full of all the real stories that make Melody such a great teacher and guide. You'll read the advice she gives to clients in her own voice—no sugar coating, no wishy-washy indecisiveness. You'll get the straight, honest answer with a good dose of empathy.

In *Diet Lies and Weight Loss Truths*, Melody has taken nearly every question that folks seeking a legitimate resource to answer their burning diet questions ask me and answers them with wisdom, humor, and practical advice. Melody's "where the rubber meets the road" writing style is concise and actionable. This is the trustworthy, evidence-based guidebook that every dieter and trainer should have at their fingertips.

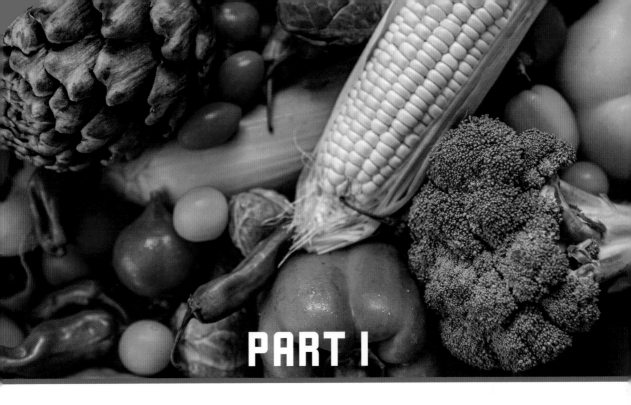

PART I

I know of a fitness chain that has a very successful business plan. They have a very, very slick social media marketing scheme that literally packs their exercise classes every day. Basically, you give them some kind of down payment, and they give you six weeks to lose 20 pounds. If you succeed in losing the weight, then you get your money back. In that six weeks, they put you on an *extremely* limited meal plan (that includes supplements they sell, of course) and beat the crap out of you in their gym five days a week. If you're not close-but-not-quite-there to the 20-pound mark toward the end of the six weeks, they limit your food much more, and even severely limit the amount of water you're allowed to drink.

A lot of people hit that 20-pound mark by the end of the six weeks. Of course they do. It's kind of hard not to when you're forced into an extreme calorie deficit like that. And I'm not gonna lie—seeing those pounds come off is exciting. It's encouraging. It's inspiring. Their friends and family will see the change, and there's a good chance some of them will jump on board, too. And so the cycle will continue.

It's a great business plan. So great, in fact, that I've seen several different gym chains in my area adopt a similar structure. There's even an exorbitantly expensive fitness certification I know of that follows this kind of plan, providing "before" and "after" photos of people who go through their x-week program, becoming suddenly glistening and muscled (I eventually learned one of the participants that the "after" photographs are generally taken when the subjects are extremely dehydrated, under extremely complimentary lighting so as to look particularly jacked. Many people are crying and exhausted at that final stage, and after their glamor shots are done, everyone goes out and eats a lot of pizza). People see the pictures and are inspired. Hell, I'm inspired just by looking at them.

Here's the problem: no one (OK, *almost* no one) is going to want to live off of steamed vegetables and tilapia forever, and few people will be able to maintain an extreme calorie deficit along with a rigorous workout schedule for an extended period of time. This is simply not a realistic plan.

The fact of the matter is, every diet works, and every diet has its pros and cons. Every diet works for one main reason: caloric deficit. What this means is that the mechanism of every diet generally comes down to eating fewer calories than you burn off. If exercise is added, then calories expended are increased as well, therefore causing even more of a deficit. To put it more simply: If I burn 1,000 calories per day, and I eat 1,500 calories a day, I'll probably put on some fat. If I burn 1,000 calories per day, and I eat 500 calories per day, I'll probably lose some fat. By the way, please don't eat only 500 calories per day. Thank you.

Some things are easier to eat a lot of than others: I can easily eat a loaf of French bread in one sitting without thinking twice about it; I've gone through a full bag of chips more times than I'd like to acknowledge; and I once ate an entire family pack of Oreo cookies in one sitting. On the other hand, I've never eaten enough broccoli to surpass the calories I burn in a day. This is why junk food is problematic. The food itself is not the problem—it's how easy it is to eat a whole bunch of it at once. So it's much easier to go way over the calories you eat in a day when you eat really tasty (i.e., hyperpalatable, for those of you who want good words to impress people at parties with) foods. Not that broccoli isn't tasty (I like it, anyway), but you're not going to find me mowing down several heads of it in one go.

So one way people can lose weight fairly easily is by replacing hyperpalatable foods (it really rolls off the tongue, doesn't it?) with other foods like veggies, 100 percent whole-grain or sprouted-grain breads, and healthy proteins. A lot of diets take a route like this—eliminating certain foods, or even entire food groups—and by default, you end up eating fewer calories.

But let's look into this in more detail.

In this section, I'm going to break down a whole lot of diets you've probably heard of, have considered trying, or have maybe even given a shot before. With each diet, I'm going to talk about why they work (spoiler alert: they pretty much all work, to some degree), problems you might experience while on these diets, and perhaps some not-so-true things you might have heard about the diet in order to get you hooked. I'll also summarize everything about each diet at the end for those of you who are short on time or patience. All of my references have been listed at the end of this book, so if you'd like to dive in and do some research of your own, that can be a good jumping-off point for you.

While you're reading this, you might think, "*Hey*. I tried X diet, and it totally worked for me when I did it!" Well, that's really the thing, isn't it—if you're not doing it anymore and your results didn't stick around, it didn't work for you. Just a little something to keep in mind.

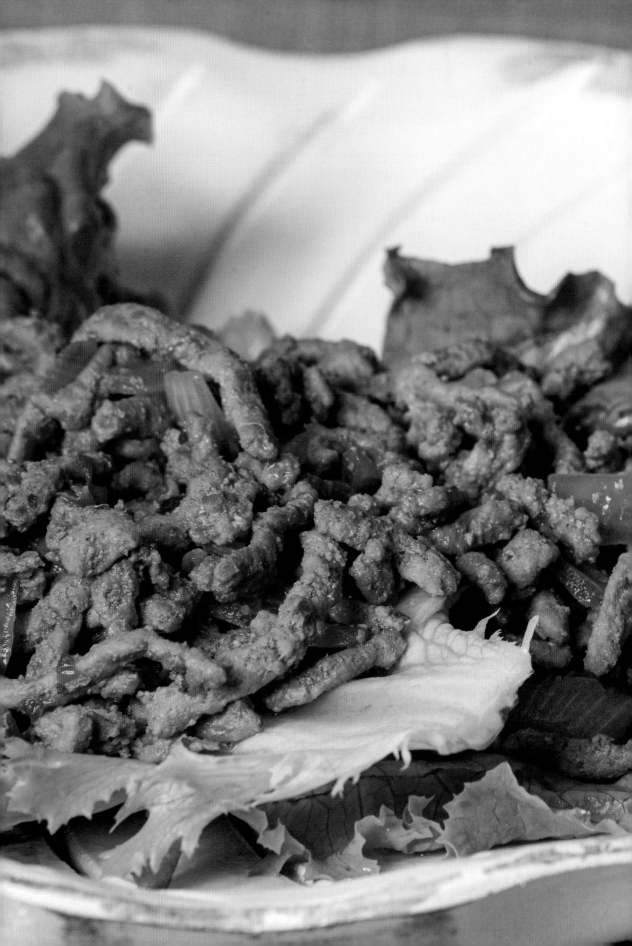

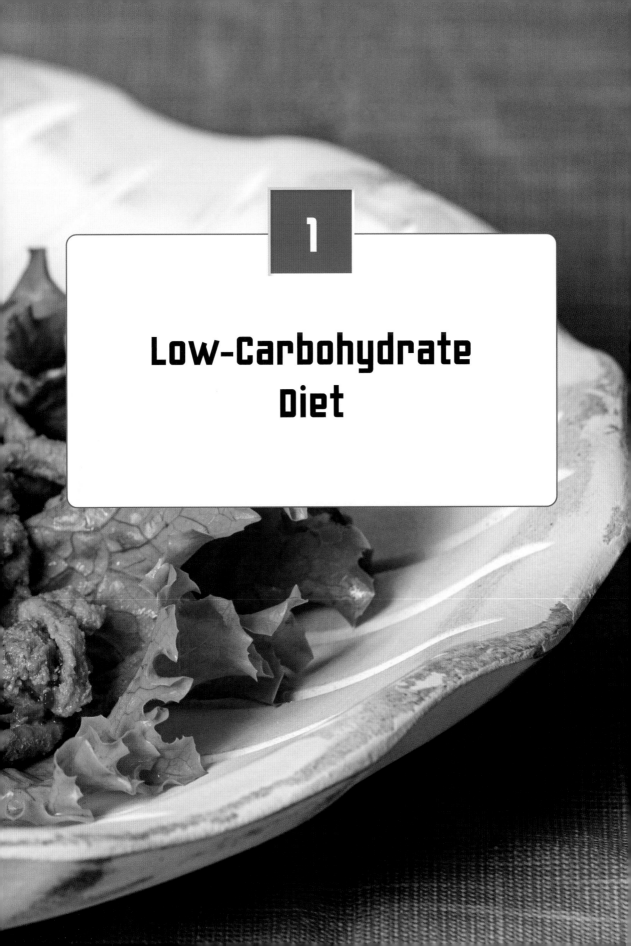

1

Low-Carbohydrate Diet

My friend Erin told me all about her experience on a low-carb diet:

"I was the kind of person who ate a lot because I rarely felt full. In my early 20s, I found out I had PCOS [polycystic ovary syndrome]. I learned that a low-carb diet could help. And I tried—oh, did I try. By the time I was 30, I weighed over 250 pounds. I stopped getting on the scale; I knew I had to do something more drastic. Over the span of a few years, I finally got down to 230 pounds. But I was hungry and miserable.

When I first switched from general low-carb (under 100 g of carbs a day) to keto (20 to 30 g of carbs), I had the opposite of the dreaded 'keto flu,' likely because I'd already started tracking what I ate and eating fewer carbs than most people. For the first time, I felt comfortably full after a meal. I was diligent. I was focused. I lost 30 pounds in less than six months—a record for me. And I finally briefly saw 'Onederland,' weighing in just under 200 pounds. It felt like I'd finally mended my broken relationship with food.

And then I ate a piece of cake at a friend's engagement party. No problem, right? I'll get right back on track. And then I had one drink at a work event a few weeks later. And then I had several drinks at a party a few days after that. And then the holidays hit, and I was so far off the keto rails, I couldn't figure out how to get back on track.

My health indicators told the story I was trying to ignore: My A1c was up from a tightly controlled 5.3 to over 9. My doctor increased my metformin dose. I gained back 20 of those 30 pounds. My life continued to have upheaval as I struggled to get back some of the control I'd had over my food choices.

However good those high-carb foods taste in my imagination, they really don't give me more than a short-term dopamine hit and longer-term negative consequences. I feel my best when I stay in low-carb eating routines, limit the scope of my food variation, and stay away from highly processed treats, even if the packaging advertises that they are low-carb or keto."

TRUTHS

When I hear people talk about losing weight, one of the first things they say is something along the lines of, "I gotta stop eating bread," or, "No more pasta for me!" Low-carb diets seem to be the current go-to for weight loss. But is a low-carb plan the panacea that everyone makes it out to be? Will eliminating sandwiches and spaghetti cause the pounds to drop off?

The low-carb lifestyle has been pushed as a weight loss miracle for some time now under different names and slightly different methods. These are some of the diets that have spawned the low-carb movement:

- Paleo
- Caveman
- Atkins
- Ketogenic (or keto)
- Protein power
- Sonoma
- Dukan

There are more, but these are some of the more popular low-carb plans.

Low-carb diets certainly are comparable to other types of diets in their effectiveness when protein and total energy intake are equated (1-3). One meta-analysis (an examination of a large group of studies on a subject) maintains that the Atkins diet was more effective than other diets when study participants were not specifically asked to stick to a particular calorie range or increase in exercise (7). Meanwhile, a 2015 study done in a metabolic ward (meaning that the researchers could observe the participants at all times and control how food and beverages were consumed, how much exercise was done, etc.) demonstrated that a low-fat diet resulted in greater fat loss than a low-carb diet, although both result in fat loss (10). The bottom line is that while low-carb diets may or may not have an edge on other diets as far as fat loss is concerned, they appear to be effective.

The main reason low-carb diets seem to work is that they are high in protein, which appears to satisfy the appetite more than carbs or fats (4-6). Whether the protein is plant- or animal-based does not seem to be an issue; either works equally well to satisfy appetite and assist in losing weight or fat (8-9). When you're not feeling hungry, you tend to eat less, which means you're eating fewer calories. And, of course, if you eat fewer calories than you burn off, then you'll lose weight.

> *While low-carb diets may or may not have an edge on other diets as far as fat loss is concerned, they appear to be effective.*

Another reason why low-carb, high-protein diets work is through something called the *thermic effect* of protein, which means that proteins burn more calories than carbs or fats (11-13). Not only that, but a high-protein diet may prevent a decline in the number of calories burned at rest better than low-protein diets (14). This means you can burn more calories for a longer period of time, even at rest. This is probably due to the increased ability to maintain the lean mass that has been attributed to a high-protein diet (14). Furthermore, there is something inherent in the ketogenic diet that curbs appetite, which, of course, leads to eating less and therefore losing weight (51).

DOWNSIDES

I know what you're thinking: "Wow! That all sounds awesome! I'm going low-carb *right now*!" Well, hold on there, Spanky. There are some downsides. There is evidence that both the satiating (i.e. hunger-satisfying) and thermal effects of protein might not last once the body adapts to a high-protein diet (13). While more research needs to be done on this, this could mean that in the long term, further strategies should be put in place to ensure continued weight loss. However, the few long-term studies that have been conducted on low-carb diets demonstrate that these diets continue to work in the long run (14).

Meanwhile, high-fat, low-carb diets, such as the Atkins diet and the ketogenic diet, may possibly raise low-density lipoproteins (LDLs) (15)—or "bad cholesterol"—which could lead to the arteries hardening if left unchecked. Although high-fat diets have some cardiovascular benefits in the short term, such as an overall reduction in obesity, a lowered risk of type 2 diabetes, and an increase in high-density lipoproteins (HDLs)—or "good cholesterol"—there is evidence showing that these benefits may not last in the long-term (16). More studies are needed on the subject of long-term health effects of these types of diets.

Another downside to low-carb diets is that they tend to exclude foods with a lot of health benefits. Whole grains, beans, fruits, and some "no-no" vegetables such as potatoes, beets, carrots, and yams are high in different nutrients that can be really beneficial. Not only that, but current evidence demonstrates that diets that are high in whole-grain foods tend to correspond to lower risks of cardiovascular disease, a lower body mass index, better digestion, and less weight gain over time (42). Cutting out these foods could be doing your body a disservice.

An extremely low-carb diet, such as the ketogenic diet, might lead to athletic performance problems. Of the studies that examine the link between ketogenic diets and athleticism, a large percentage have no control group, are poorly designed, or have significant potential bias in their reporting. While more research is needed on this subject, the current evidence demonstrates that ketogenic diets perform about as well as, or slightly less than, high-carb diets for endurance and strength (43), and this may interfere with the ability to gain muscle mass (44). None of the current studies show any athletic advantage of the ketogenic diet.

The biggest downside to low-carb, high-protein diets is compliance (14). It is just not easy to maintain such a highly restricted diet, and a lot of people drop out. However, if you can stick with it, and if you make smart choices, a low-carb, high-protein diet will be a very effective way to lose weight.

LIES

I've seen a lot of pretty shady statements about various low-carb diets. Let's just go ahead and nip those in the bud right now.

Bacon

Bacon is not a magical health food. I know this seems like common sense, but bacon is *everywhere* and well entrenched in many popular low-carb plans. Everything is suddenly wrapped in it, covered in it, slathered in it, and even cooked in bacon grease. However, there does appear to be a link between processed, red, and cured meats and cancer, heart disease, and all-cause mortality (20-21).

When looking at the results of these studies, it's important to note that many of them are epidemiological studies, which means that a certain population was studied, and elements of their diet or lifestyle were examined to see if a relationship to the thing being studied might exist. So while consuming read meat and processed meat certainly seems to be linked to these conditions, we cannot say for sure that they—and not some other lifestyle factor (or a combination of these foods and specific lifestyle factors)—are the cause. The issue might also be related to the way the meats were prepared; if they were prepared a different way, then a different result would occur. We also cannot definitively tell from these studies that a specific "bad" dose of meat exists. How much meat would cause these issues? If you eat less meat than that, will you not get those issues? Despite such holes in the currently existing studies, the evidence demonstrates a pretty reliable link, particularly in the case of processed meat and cured meat, so it's best not to load up on them.

Coconut Oil

Coconut oil is also not a magical health food. The studies that led to this conclusion generally looked at populations who eat a lot of coconut and also have low instances of heart disease and overall lower mortality rates (17). However, the people who were studied also live in areas of the South Pacific that generally eat a traditional pescatarian, whole-foods diet with no processed foods. It also doesn't influence the discussion about diets. This comes in major contrast to a typical Western diet, which tends to be high in processed foods and low in fruits, vegetables, and fish. When considered within the context of a Westernized population, coconut oil doesn't appear to be more beneficial than any other saturated fat and in large amounts could potentially raise the risk of heart disease (18-21).

Contrary to some common claims, whether or not coconut oil can help with weight loss has *not* been confirmed (22-24). The existing studies on this are mostly very small, poorly designed, and biased. Coconut oil is about 60 percent medium-chain triglycerides (MCTs). While some studies have published evidence on the benefits of MCTs, this is definitely a gray area that needs a lot more research before any conclusions can be made.

The Skinny on Saturated Fat

Let's tag on to the theme of bacon and coconut oil. Many low-carb gurus tout the benefits of saturated fats, explaining that they are not harmful to health like we always believed. When the sources of saturated fats and other lifestyle and dietary aspects are not considered, studies do demonstrate that they are, in fact, pretty benign (25-27).

The issue becomes muddier, though, when we consider what the saturated fat is replaced with. A Western diet, for example, tends to be high in refined carbs, trans fats, and sugars. If you compare a diet high in saturated fats to a Westernized diet, like the one I just mentioned, the saturated fats without junk foods will demonstrate a lower risk of heart problems and other diseases (26-29). But when a diet high in saturated fats is compared to one high in monounsaturated or polyunsaturated fats like omega-3 and omega-6, the risk of disease is much higher for saturated fats (26-27). When saturated fats are replaced with unprocessed, complex carbs like vegetables, beans, and whole grains, the risks also decrease (28-29). Saturated fat coming from milk and cheese may lower the risk of heart disease more than that coming from meat, but unsaturated fats still reign superior to either kind of saturated fat (29-30). Replacing animal-based saturated fats with protein—particularly plant protein—also appears to possibly reduce the risk of heart disease (29-30). Furthermore, the body naturally produces its own saturated fats; it is unnecessary to consume them. The bottom line is that there is no biological need to eat saturated fats; when it comes down to consuming them, it's not just about reducing saturated fats—it's about replacing them with something healthier.

Weight Loss Versus Fat Loss

One issue with many studies is that they concentrate on *weight* loss rather than *fat* loss. These two things are not quite the same. Your body's weight does not reflect your body's composition. (I've seen my own weight fluctuate up to 10 lb in a day, depending on what I ate and what time of the month it was.) Weight loss on a low-carb diet can often be explained by water loss—carbs are converted to glycogen in the body, and glycogen stores a couple of grams of water along with it. When your carb intake is low, your body starts to use stored glycogen as fuel, which means it will shed the stored water along with it. It's a pretty cool trick I've used for powerlifting if I needed to make weight for a competition. The week before the competition, I'd cut way down on carbs. I'd be grumpy and miserable, but by weigh-in time, I'd be a few pounds lighter. Then I'd eat a sandwich, and all would be well again. That isn't to say that low-carb diets don't cause body fat loss; the available information shows that they do, comparably to other popular diets. But any edge in weight loss might be explained by water loss, and this water loss phenomenon does not last for the long term.

▪ Wrap It Up

- Low-carb diets appear to be about as effective as other diets for weight loss when calories are equated.
- Whether or not these diets are healthful in the long term is unclear.
- A lot more high-quality, unbiased, and long-term studies are needed on the subject.
- According to current evidence, saturated fats should be reduced *and* replaced by polyunsaturated fats, healthy carbs, and proteins (particularly plant protein) in order to maintain optimal health. What replaces them is key.

Greek
Yogurt
NONFAT
Mango

Grade A
Blended

0%
MILKFAT

NET WT. 5.3 OZ (150g)

2

Low-Fat Diet

My friend Dave Barry, former AAU Mr. America and NABBA Mr. USA, shared with me his various experiences on different diets, including the low-fat diet:

"I've experimented with various types of diets such as low-fat (LF), low-carb (LC), and a ketogenic (low-carb/high-fat [LCHF]) diet between 1984 and 2020. At multiple times, I used each dietary regime between 20 weeks and several years while implementing each plan rigidly, along with four to five days of weight training a week, and three to six days of cardiovascular conditioning a week.

Initially, both the LC and LCHF diets resulted in more significant weight loss as compared to the LF diet during the first three to four weeks. However, after the first month, I saw similar weight loss between all the different dietary plans assuming similar 'net calories per day.'

Each of the plans got me to the endpoint I desired. I ultimately chose to stick with a LF diet because it allowed for the most variety among food groups. Additionally, the LC diet was high in protein, which, over time, appeared to cause intermittent bouts of constipation possibly due to lower fiber, since fruits and complex carbohydrates were limited. Finally, the LCHF diet didn't seem to provide me the same energy levels while performing high-intensity weight training as compared to the LF diet. Consequently, I've found the LF diet to have more variety as well as provide more usable energy for weight training, making it easier for me to adhere to in the long term."

TRUTHS

When it comes to weight loss, low-fat diets seem to perform about as well as other diets do when calories are matched (meaning they probably aren't dripping with fat-free cookies and rubbery fatless cheese products) (2, 35-37). Energy balance is the key—I cannot overstate this enough.

> *Unfortunately, the general idea—*
> *and I was guilty of this as well—*
> *was that if food was fat free,*
> *you could have a lot of it, and*
> *it wouldn't "count" (31). That is*
> *simply not how energy balance*
> *works, unfortunately.*

Let's set aside the problems with chowing down on low-fat munchies for a moment. Another issue with low-fat diets is that, when cutting out the "bad" fats, you are also cutting out the "good" fats that will likely help your heart. As mentioned in the low-carb section, replacing saturated fats with processed carbs like white flour and sugary snacks is as bad or worse for your heart than the saturated fats (26-29, 38-39). The best option is to replace at least a portion of saturated fats with polyunsaturated fats such as omega-3 and omega-6 (26-27), as well as whole grains, fruits, and proteins (28-30).

In a low-fat diet, you won't get much in the way of omega-3s or omega-6s. In an extremely low-fat diet (less than 10 percent of calories from fat), you might even end up with an essential fatty acid deficiency—which can lead to problems such as rashes, hair loss, loss of hair color, problems with wound healing, and immune issues—and can even put you at risk for Alzheimer's disease and dementia (40-41).

LIES

Growing up, my dad struggled with obesity and heart issues, and I remember my mom constantly trying to curtail his intake of fatty foods. So we had a fridge pantry full of all kinds of fat-free things. We had fat-free cheese, skim milk, and tons of these chocolate cookies called Snackwell's, which led to an incident in which the dog broke into the pantry and ate several boxes of the aforementioned cookies, leading to panicked calls to the vet's office, leading to the realization that the dog had a steel-plated stomach and was immune to being affected by eating several boxes of Snackwell's . . . but I digress.

Anyway, the low-fat diet phenomenon was all the rage in the 1980s and '90s. It emerged from findings from the 1940s and beyond that high-fat diets corresponded with high cholesterol levels, which was a potential red flag for heart disease risk (31). Dietary fat in the '80s was the Devil at the time; it was considered to be the cause of obesity, heart problems, and even cancer (31). Major magazines and newspapers touted the greatness of the low-fat diet. And with this movement came a plethora of fat-free treats in which fat was replaced by sugar in order to make it palatable. The result was snacks that were similar in calories to the original but very high in sugar—although fat free.

That fat-free label made a lot of people very, very rich. I remember eating fat-free Entenmann's cakes and cookies with my bestie Robyn—the whole box between the two of us—and we thought it was fine because of that fat-free label. Leagues of people felt the same. In fact, companies could even purchase an "American Heart Association Seal of Approval" for their products, and many did (31-32). The main issue here, besides the obvious one of being able to actually *purchase* a "heart-healthy" label from a supposedly reputable agency, was that the labels tended to go on processed snack foods instead of foods like fresh fruits and veggies (31-32). The list of over 600 labeled products included Frosted Flakes, Cocoa Krispies, and Froot Loops (32).

Another big, glaring issue here was that a low-fat diet had never been *proven* to prevent heart disease, just as a high-fat diet had never been *proven* to increase the risk. Again, studies were based on epidemiological evidence, so the culprit was nebulous. Another issue was that the studies from the mid-'80s were performed on middle-aged men only (31), so a huge portion of the population was not studied. What we basically had was a nationwide health recommendation based on shady evidence from a fraction of the population.

What ended up happening was, despite everyone jumping on the low-fat bandwagon, obesity rates continued to rise steadily. In fact, between 1980 and 2000, United States obesity rates for the aged-20-to-74 population rose from around 10 percent for men and around 15 percent for women to close to 30 percent for men and about 35 percent for women (33-34). Unfortunately, the general idea—and I was guilty of this as well—was that if food was fat-free, you could have a lot of it, and it wouldn't "count" (31). That is simply not how energy balance works. As a result, an overabundance of calories helped lead to an overabundance of weight gain.

At the same time, interestingly, coronary disease decreased significantly (34). However, this was largely due to advances in medical science, a reduction in smoking habits, and an increase in physical activity (34). Low-fat diets full of processed snack foods likely did not play much of a role.

■ Wrap It Up

- Low-fat diets were falsely believed to lead to weight loss and a lowered risk of heart disease.
- A low-fat diet, if matched in calories to other diets, has similar weight loss capabilities. The key is the energy balance.
- If fat intake is too low, serious health problems can occur.

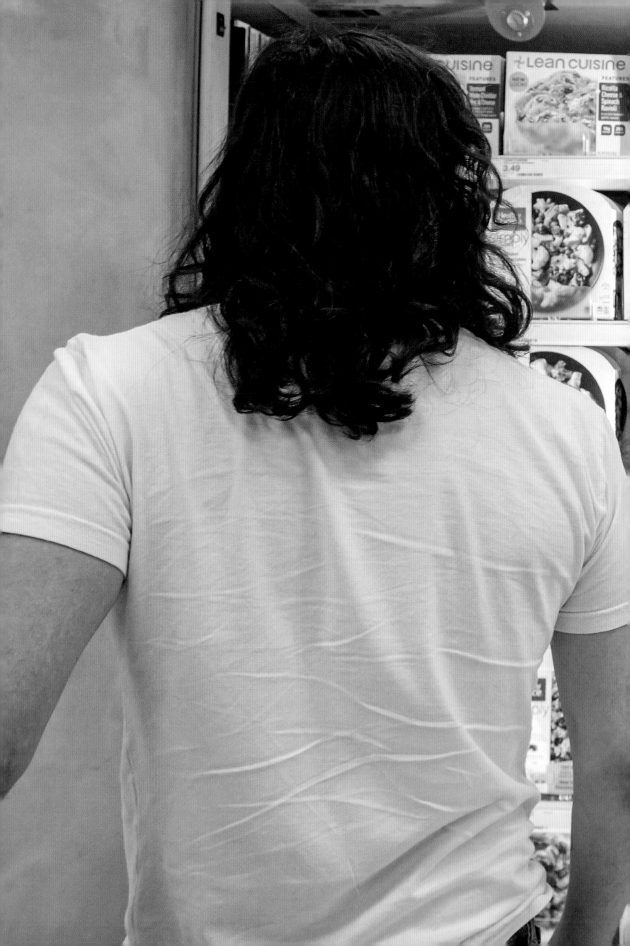

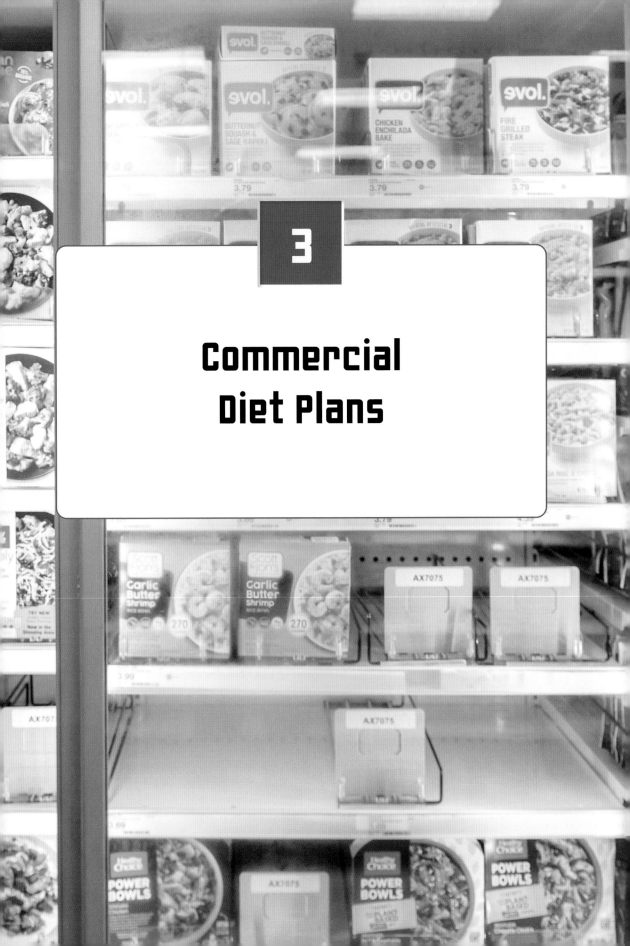

3

Commercial Diet Plans

A friend of mine shared his experience on one prepackaged meal plan:

"My goal was to drop 20 pounds and go on a date with a model. I ended up doing both.

Physically, I did lose the weight fast. I wasn't hungry that much. The bars gave me epic diarrhea most days, which they said was 'the body detoxing,' which is utter crap (no pun intended).

I was on the diet for six weeks, give or take. I was 185 pounds when I started and got down to 165 pounds and one jean size smaller. I stopped because it's expensive and I made my goal. After that, I started being less careful with what I ate, ate more treats and pastries, more carbs and potatoes and . . . it crept back on. I maintained 175 pounds for a while. I'm 190 pounds now, down from 195. Cutting carbs and going keto-ish."

My friend Susie also shared her experience with the same program:

"Okay, for me it was a good plan. I am actually doing it right now since I went off the rails when the whole shelter in place started and gained a few more pounds than I am comfortable with. I lost about 50 pounds last year. There is more than one plan with it, but the main weight loss one is where you eat five of their prepackaged products and one meal that is protein and low-carb veggies. You used to have to get the program from a doctor, but now you get it from 'health coaches.'

The first few days were hard—not going to lie. I drank a lot of water and had some sugar-free Jell-O or pickles to help me get by.

The one plus of their products is that they have probiotics and all the vitamins and good stuff you need—in fact, my blood work after being on the program was better than it had been in 10 years. I was able to donate blood for the first time in years as well because my anemia was no longer an issue.

I am a binge eater and an emotional eater, and I have such an effed-up relationship with food that having the structure of exactly what I am eating and when was beneficial for me. Another facet of the program is the 'health coaching' and support you get. A 'health coach' is basically someone who has successfully worked the program and now they help others. And my coach is hooked up with an online Facebook support group. Support is important.

Now, the prepackaged food can get expensive, so they give you substitutions, which are high-protein, low-carb, and low-fat foods you can eat instead. But you still eat five a day and one meal.

A diet is only sustainable if you plan on following it to the end. Once you finish losing weight, there is a transition where it helps you to start incorporating regular foods into your diet, such as whole grains and fruits. If you do not go through the transition and just start eating the way you did then, yeah, you can gain weight quickly, but that is the case with any weight loss, no matter what program or method you used to lose the weight.

I have done multiple weight loss programs, bought all the workout gear, and had bariatric surgery in 2000. But it is only in the last five years that I have had the most success, and that is with having a physical job and really being mindful. When I took time off in 2018, I hired a personal trainer for seven months to keep me accountable. The support component of the program is a plus for me."

TRUTHS

Weight Watchers, Jenny Craig, Nutrisystem, SlimFast, and similar diets fall in the category of commercial diet plans. More recently, meal delivery services such as Blue Apron, Purple Carrot, and the like might also fall into this category, even if they are not specifically weight loss programs.

> *If you follow the plans the way they are designed, you cannot overeat, and therefore you will not go beyond a certain number of calories per day.*

Commercial diet plans essentially limit the amount of food that you eat through a number of techniques—points systems, boxed foods (portion limitations), pre-portioned ingredients, and so on. If you follow the plans the way they are designed, you cannot overeat, and therefore you will not go beyond a certain number of calories per day. In the case of Blue Apron-type companies, the meals themselves may not be designated low-calorie per se, but they are portion-controlled and generally stay within a reasonable number of calories per meal, so they may inadvertently contribute to weight loss. Commercial diet plans appear to work about as well as other named diet plans, whether low-carb or low-fat, if the diets are followed (2). Of the most popular diets studied, Weight Watchers, seems to be the most cost-effective, as it does not include the cost of food (47).

DOWNSIDES

Unfortunately, most people do not seem to stick to commercial diet plans. Current evidence demonstrates that a large percentage of people who start a diet like Weight Watchers or Jenny Craig fall off the wagon within the first year (45). Plans are often not cost-effective (46); depend on packaged foods that, let's face it, almost no one wants to eat forever; or use other methods such as liquid meal replacements or very low-calorie strategies that are simply not sustainable for a large percentage of people embarking on these programs.

Once again, a problem with current research is that many available studies are poorly designed, lack a control group, have significant bias, are too small, or do not assess the long-term effects of these diets. In addition, dropout rates are extremely high for many of the studies examining commercial diets, so it is difficult to say how they might affect people health-wise in the long run.

As far as meal kit delivery services such as Blue Apron and Purple Carrot go, there is virtually no research currently available about their impact on weight loss. However, one analysis from an environmental perspective demonstrates that meal kits save about 33 percent of energy and emissions compared to purchasing groceries from the store. On the downside, they produce about 3.7 pounds more packaging per meal (48). Therefore, meal kits have somewhat of an environmental edge compared to grocery shopping, but they have some work to do when it comes to excess packaging. As far as my own personal (completely nonscientific) opinion on meal kits: Most of them use high-quality ingredients and significantly more vegetables than the average American tends to eat. They have the potential to teach and encourage more people to cook at home, which can be a major plus, and they are inherently portion controlled. Depending on how often you eat out or shop for groceries, they can potentially be cost-prohibitive. It may be worth calculating the costs of your weekly meals out and comparing them to the cost of meal kits to determine if this is a good option for you.

Lies

Commercial diets are notorious for using celebrity spokespeople to advertise their products and sometimes they use a random person with a name like "Lisa M." and add, in small print, "*results not typical." The problem is that they don't tell you whether or not these people stuck to the diet for the long term. Sometimes you won't even notice, because a representative who gains the weight back will be replaced quickly with a new successful one, and that's the one you'll concentrate on. It's important to remember that a diet is only successful if you stick to it. The spokespeople may or may not have been able to stick to these diets in the long term. The bottom line is that you shouldn't use spokespeople as definitive proof of a diet; it's only going to work for as long as you're able to follow it consistently.

Wrap It Up

Basically, if you can afford the cost of one of these programs and are able to stick to it ongoing, chances are that you'll lose weight on the diet, at least in the short term. Whether or not those results will continue for the long term is not conclusive.

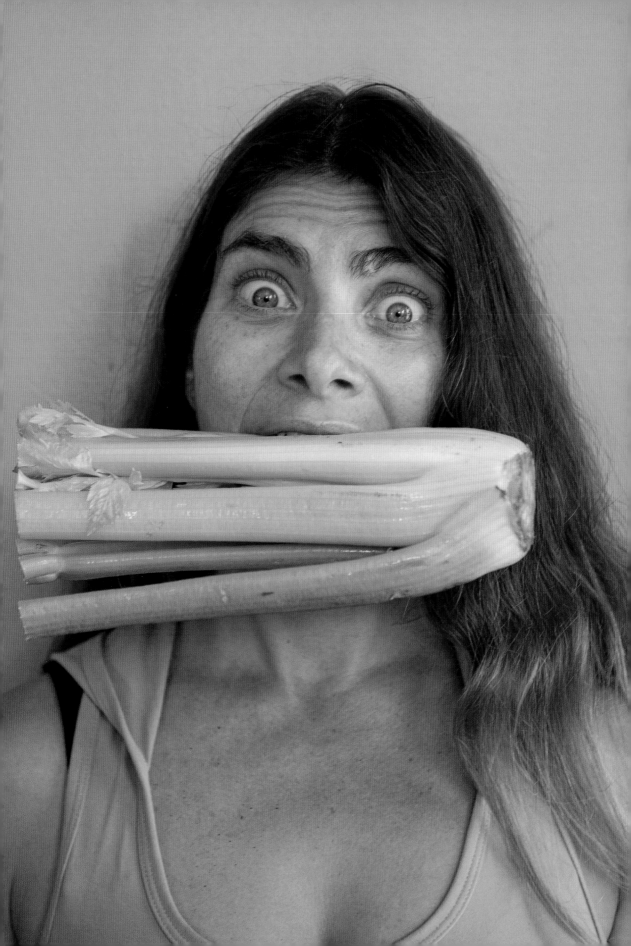

4

Vegan Diet

Icelandic powerlifter Hulda Waage shared with me her experience with veganism as a strength athlete:

"I felt it straight away in my strength journey that getting stronger physically meant I became stronger mentally. The difference was huge. I controlled my emotions better, and I was more capable of standing up for myself and others in situations in which I had just felt unworthy before.

The same thing happened when I went vegan. I felt so aligned with my emotions. Standing my ground and living my beliefs made me mentally stronger.

I felt a huge relief: being true to myself. The mental aspect of strength is the biggest part of it all—to be stronger you have to believe you can and that you are.

The physical benefits I felt when going vegan were there too. My digestion got so much better. My stomach wasn't as heavy. I had much more energy.

This means I can train more and recover faster as long as I mostly choose whole foods. My body feels good; it is stronger, and my mentality is stronger too. The only regret that I have is not going vegan sooner."

TRUTHS

There are a lot of reasons why people go vegan. I have personally been vegan since 2000 for moral reasons (I'm a major animal lover), and this is the driving force for many vegans. Some do it for environmental reasons, while others believe it will improve their health. And, of course, there are those who go vegan because they believe it will help them lose weight. But is veganism really a weight loss magic bullet?

Plant-based diets do seem to be correlated with successful weight loss (49-50), and there is even some promising (but inconclusive) evidence that a vegan diet might be useful in reducing HbA1c levels, which is a significant marker of diabetes risk (52). Observational and interventional studies consistently conclude that diets that are high in vegetables, fruits, and whole grains tend to correlate to lower body weight than the diet used as the control; however, randomized, controlled studies at this point have not shown conclusive evidence that an increase in plant foods alone makes a difference in body weight (53-54). In one meta-analysis of randomized controlled studies, vegetarian diets seemed to have an advantage for weight loss, and vegan diets had an advantage over vegetarian diets; however, the results are inconclusive (54).

Now, this is all well and good, but there are some points to consider here. As mentioned earlier, observational, interventional, and epidemiological studies cannot really say, "Yeah, veggie diets are definitely the key to weight loss." There are just too many outside factors that could affect the results. Furthermore, none of the randomized studies appeared to have equated calories between control groups and plant-based groups. Some of them gave calorie guidelines, but none equated calories, so we don't know if the difference was due to the contents of the diet itself or the number of calories consumed. In addition, none of the studies controlled or monitored the food intake, which means that the subjects kept diaries or otherwise self-reported their own data. When left to their own devices, people tend to overreport exercise and underreport food intake by a significant amount, leading to major inaccuracies in data (55-56).

A pretty fair conclusion to make is that vegans and vegetarians, as a general rule, tend to eat fewer calories than omnivores. Vegetables are dense in nutrients but relatively low in calories (depending, of course, on how they're prepared), so a diet high in veggies and other plant foods is generally a low-calorie diet. Of course, plenty of not-so-healthy foods are, or can be made, vegan—from chips and fries to candies, ice cream, cookies, donuts, and pastries, vegan junk foods abound. These types of foods are extremely easy to eat a lot of. So while a whole foods-based, heavy-on-the-veggies vegan diet can be conducive to weight loss due to its lower calorie count, a vegan diet with large amounts of fried and sugary foods may not be so great for the waistline. Once again, it really comes down to calories.

LIES

There are, unfortunately, a lot of lies told about the vegan diet, both on the side of omnivores and on the side of vegans. As an example of the lies on the vegan side, I'd like to show you an article I recently wrote:

Ladies and gentlemen, you're being lied to.

It may be subtle, and it may be wrapped in an earnest-looking package, but truly, you are being lied to, and it's time these lies were called out.

Let me explain.

Not long ago, I submitted a request to write an article for a popular vegan magazine. The response I received was . . . enlightening. This was part of the magazine editor's very lengthy response to my request:

> We do not recommend books with this sort of a message, which is contrary to everything that we teach in the pages of _____ Magazine. . . . We publish articles in every issue that enforce the important message that going vegan is not difficult. . . .

When she says "this sort of a message," she is responding to my having written extensively about the fact that vegans may need to supplement certain nutrients that aren't found in the vegan diet or that aren't absorbed as well. So what she's saying is that this magazine will only support information that portrays the vegan diet as one that does not really require any extra work or attention. This is a dangerous idea, and one that could get people pretty sick.

The editor goes on to say this:

> There is no substitute for doing your own scientific research. The sources that we rely on are large peer-reviewed studies like the Framingham study. The folks we rely on are nutritional scientists like T. Colin Campbell, Pamela Popper, and The Loma Linda Hospital and Nutritional Research Center in California.

In short, she will only consider data from studies and researchers whom she agrees with. There's a word for this practice: cherry-picking. Scientific research should not be a process of looking for studies that confirm your bias. Not only that, but it's also important to look at the quality of a study, how many other studies have found similar results, who the sponsor of a study is, and so on. Cherry-picking provides biased information that can lead to not-so-accurate conclusions. When you only have part of the information, there's a good chance you'll make some pretty poor choices.

Unfortunately, this editor is not the only one using half-truths to push an agenda, and it isn't only found within the vegan community. You'll see it in documentaries, books, magazines, newspapers, and, yes, sometimes even in scientific studies. It is therefore so important to be aware of your sources. Just because someone is a doctor with a bestselling book, for instance, does not mean that that person has the right answers to your nutrition questions. A fitness professional with a great body and a huge social media following isn't necessarily knowledgeable about biomechanics. Being the loudest one in the room doesn't equate to knowing the most.

It looks like bad information is everywhere. So what's a person to do? Here are two questions I like to consider first:

- Does this source have a particular agenda to push? (This in and of itself doesn't necessarily mean that they're not a good source, but it should raise a few flags.)

- Does this source have a product to sell?

Georgetown University published a pretty handy list of questions you can ask yourself about information you find on the Internet: www.library.georgetown.edu/tutorials/research-guides/evaluating-internet-content.

Scientific American also published a good article about wading through the information web and scientific research: http://blogs.scientificamerican.com/guest-blog/finding-good-information-on-the-internet.

Giving only part of the story is a dangerous practice, and it quite frankly stinks that we live in a world in which so much pseudoscience, misinformation, and half-truths are so easily spread. The good news is that you can be your own advocate. You're being lied to—but you can help call out the nonsense.

> *Veganism, while potentially healthier in comparison to many other lifestyles (depending on how it's approached), is not a cure-all. It also does require an understanding of nutrition and some supplementation or use of fortified foods, particularly for athletes.*

So, yes, half-truths and lies are told on the vegan side to try to convert more people. Veganism, while potentially healthier in comparison to many other lifestyles (depending on how it's approached), is not a cure-all. It also requires an understanding of nutrition and some supplementation or use of fortified foods, particularly for athletes.

On the other side of the coin, there is plenty of anti-vegan propaganda that tries to convince people *not* to go vegan. Some of those lies include the following.

"There Is No Such Thing as a Healthy Vegan"

I could just say that I am proof that this is untrue, and I could give tons of examples of other vegans who are clearly robustly strong and healthy, but that wouldn't be very scientific of me, now would it? So here's some science for you:

• The Academy of Nutrition and Dietetics and the Italian Society of Human Nutrition agree that a well-designed vegan diet is perfectly healthy and may even provide a healthy edge over other diets (62, 64). The following is a direct quote from the Academy of Nutrition and Dietetics (62):

It is the position of the Academy of Nutrition and Dietetics that appropriately planned vegetarian, including vegan, diets are healthful, nutritionally adequate, and may provide health benefits *for the prevention and treatment of certain diseases. These diets are appropriate for all stages of the life cycle, including pregnancy, lactation, infancy, childhood, adolescence, older adulthood, and for athletes. Plant-based diets are more environmentally sustainable than diets rich in animal products because they use fewer natural resources and are associated with much less environmental damage. Vegetarians and vegans are at a reduced risk of certain health conditions, including ischemic heart disease, type 2 diabetes, hypertension, certain types of cancer, and obesity. Low intakes of saturated fat and high intakes of vegetables, fruits, whole grains, legumes, soy products, nuts, and seeds (all rich in fiber and phytochemicals) are characteristics of vegetarian and vegan diets that produce lower total and low-density lipoprotein cholesterol levels and better serum glucose control. These factors contribute to reduction of chronic disease. Vegans need reliable sources of vitamin B_{12} such as fortified foods or supplements.*

The Italian Society of Human Nutrition recommends a B_{12} supplement and protein intake significantly higher than that recommended for omnivores (64).

- The German Nutrition Society (GNS), however, has a different opinion (63):

With a pure plant-based diet it is difficult or impossible to attain an adequate supply of some nutrients. The most critical nutrient is B_{12}... The DGE does not recommend a vegan diet for pregnant women, lactating women, infants, children, or adolescents.

Essentially, the GNS response recommends supplementing the vegan diet with fortified foods and other nutritional supplements in order to meet all nutritional needs, which is a fair assessment. The GNS recommends getting advice from a nutritionist and getting regular checkups to ensure that nutritional needs are being met on a vegan diet. This is fair advice that I recommend as well; I would, however, recommend this for anyone, vegan or not.

Regarding veganism and pregnancy, there is very little conclusive evidence on the subject. Existing evidence is not very high quality and isn't consistent enough to demonstrate benefits or problems with veganism during pregnancy. There does seem to be a small correlation with low birth weight and veganism, but several studies show no such issue (65-66). The authors of one large review on the subject concluded that as long as the mother is careful to meet all vitamin, mineral, and trace element needs, pregnant women and their babies should be safe following a vegan diet (66).

One meta-analysis found a correlation between vegan diets and positive health effects such as lowered risk of ischemic heart disease and total cancer risk (57). However, no significantly lowered risk of specific cancers, risk of death from all diseases, or risk of total cardio- and cerebrovascular disease is currently noted (57).

In another study in which the quality of food was accounted for, a "healthy" plant-based diet (i.e., low consumption of processed, junk-type, and convenience foods and high consumption of whole foods, fruits, and vegetables) demonstrated a 5 percent lower risk of all-cause mortality over an "unhealthy" vegetarian or omnivorous diet (i.e., higher in processed foods, animal products, added sugars, etc.) in women but not in men (58).

In an analysis of two large cohort studies, substituting plant proteins for animal proteins was associated with a lower all-cause mortality risk, and animal protein consumption was associated with a higher risk of cardiovascular disease than plant protein consumption (59).

According to a recent meta-analysis, a vegan diet is about as effective as other dietary approaches to lowering blood pressure (61). While vegan diets done correctly can help lower blood pressure, there are also less restrictive ways to do this that will work just as well.

Once again, when we look at these studies, we also have to realize a few things. First of all, they are mostly epidemiological studies, which, as I've been saying ad nauseum, can't really point to a definite cause to the effect in question. Second, there are some nebulous terms used in many of these studies: *vegetarian* and *plant-based*, to name two of them. Vegan diets may fall within the definition of both categories, but neither of them specifically refers to vegans. Studies specifically looking at vegans are much rarer. The moral of the story is that we need a lot more well-designed, large studies on a variety of different populations to get a better understanding of the vegan diet and its relationship to human health. That being said, current evidence suggests that it is entirely possible to be in excellent health as a vegan, provided all nutritional needs are met through diet, supplementation, and fortified foods.

"Vegans Are Weak and Can't Build Muscle"

The myth of the weak, skinny vegan is rampant. Comedians throw it in their acts, and recently a popular podcast tried to call out vegan strongman Patrik Baboumian, saying great strongmen cannot possibly be vegan. Even in my small corner of the strength world, I've been accused more than once of using steroids (ehm, no) or tricks to perform the old-time strongman feats of strength I like to practice.

There are plenty of examples of elite vegan athletes (Venus Williams, Scott Jurek, Jermain Defoe, Barny Du Plessis, Tia Blanco, Heather Mills, Alex Dargatz, Rob Bigwood, and many, many more), which demonstrates that even at the very top level of their sport, vegans can, in fact, be extremely strong, muscular, and athletic. However, there are very few studies that have examined vegan athletic performance in comparison to that of omnivores. Among the studies that currently exist, a vegan or vegetarian diet on its own does not seem to negatively affect athletic performance (60, 67-70), although one study demonstrated that while performance was not affected by a vegetarian diet (this one was looking at a lacto-ovo diet, not a vegan diet, so keep that in mind), muscle mass was greater in meat eaters than in vegetarians (69). In another study comparing a soy protein source to a beef protein source in older males consuming a lacto-ovo vegetarian diet, a difference in muscle mass was not seen (70). So, while the jury is still out, it does appear quite possible that meat is not a prerequisite for strength and performance. That being said, vegan athletes will have different nutritional needs from the average person. But that is fodder for another book. Or (shameless self-promotion) you can check out my article on the subject entitled "Nutritional Considerations for the Vegan Female Athlete" published in the *Strength and Conditioning Journal*.

The moral of the story is this: Lots of lies are told about the vegan diet on both sides of the line. Be careful who you listen to.

PLANT-BASED DIETS

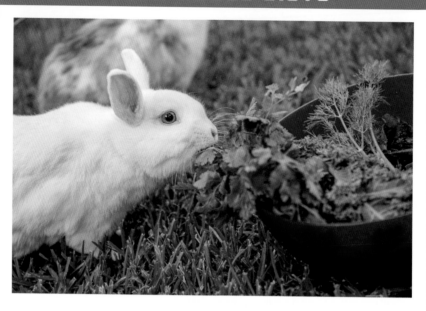

The term *plant-based* is a big buzz phrase these days. The problem is, no one really knows what it means because it doesn't have a concrete definition. It's not necessarily vegan, and it's not necessarily even vegetarian. It seems to imply that most of the diet (what percentage, we don't know) comes from plant foods, or at least nonanimal sources.

Does It Work?

Good question. It depends. There's a good chance that a plant-based diet is going to have a lot more whole foods and vegetables in it and fewer junk foods. If that is the case, then by nature of eliminating the foods people tend to overeat, it could certainly help with weight loss. However, plant-based foods aren't always healthy, aren't always whole foods-based, and aren't always low-calorie. I could eat nothing but Junior Mints and movie popcorn all day and technically stay plant based. And I'm pretty sure I could eat enough Junior Mints and movie popcorn to surpass my daily calories before lunchtime.

There is also the whole foods plant-based diet, which is a little clearer—it emphasizes eating mainly foods that are minimally processed: lots of veggies, whole grains, beans, legumes, and healthy plant-based fats. That's all great. And, again, you could lose weight on such a diet, as long as you're eating fewer calories than you're burning off, which could be easier to do when you stick to a minimally processed diet.

If we can't define a diet's parameters, then we really can't say much about it. The success of the diet depends on how you choose to follow it. The premise is good, though—eat more plants, eat less junk. Absolutely. Do that.

■ Wrap It Up

Vegan diets may contribute to weight loss, but (surprise!) it comes down to how many calories you're eating in relation to how many you're burning off. Vegan diets can be perfectly healthy, may provide some great health effects, and do not appear to negatively (or positively) affect athletic performance. The caveat with all of this is "when done correctly." It is important to ensure that any nutritional holes within the vegan diet are addressed through proper dietary planning, supplementation, and fortified foods.

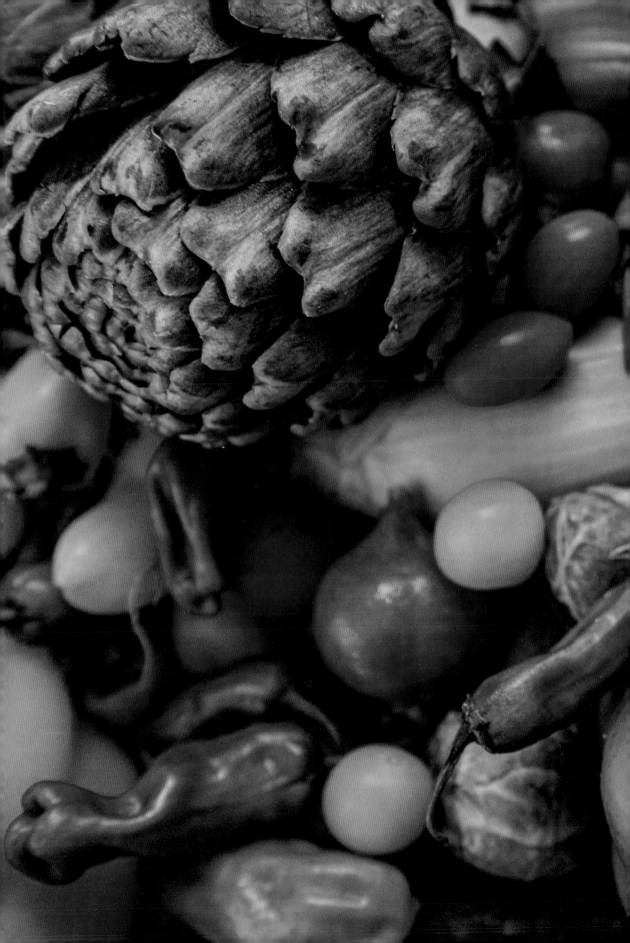

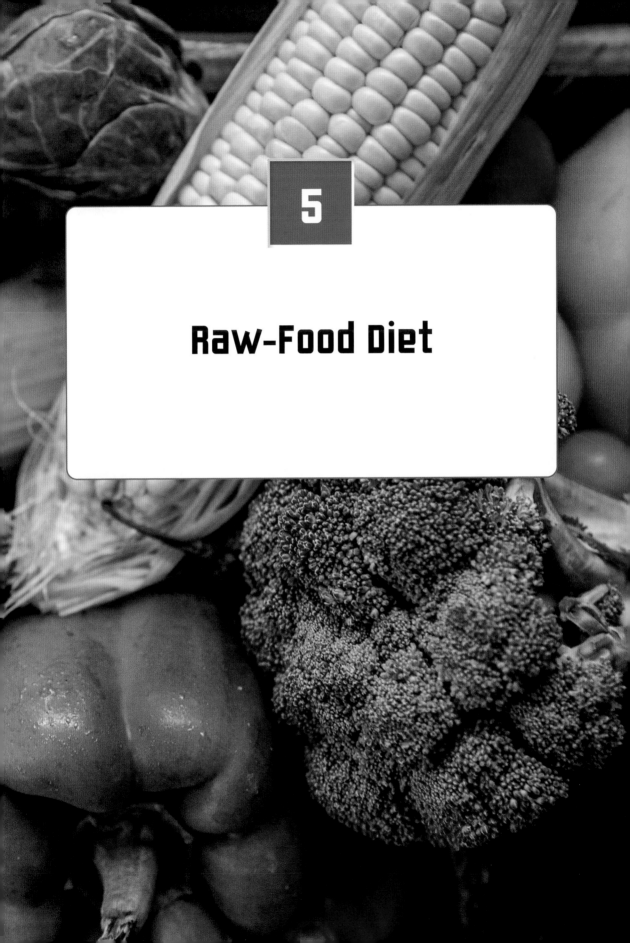

5

Raw-Food Diet

My friend Shy shared her experience on the raw diet: "I was first interested in eating raw after visiting a raw restaurant and discovering how much I loved their desserts. I was already vegan at the time and was concerned about how cooking at high heat was denaturing some of the nutrients I was hoping to get from the healthy foods I was preparing. I was already familiar with the tough cell walls of certain fibrous plants, like tomatoes and kale, for example, that require a lot of chewing and dismantling to truly benefit from.

Eating raw seemed like a perfect balance of both worlds if I incorporated a good mixer, dehydrator, and finely chopping my veggies. I did not notice any particular change in my energy, weight, skin, or hair at the time. I loved the foods I ate and got creative with the things that I ate. I was involved in long-distance cycling and resistance training at the time and found that I had to buy and consume a lot more groceries to satiate myself.

I became discouraged and eventually quit because it took too much preparation for my busy lifestyle. Fast carbs like bread and pasta were cheaper and easier snacks. A small slice of chicken breast was also faster, simpler, and could keep me full longer. I honestly was much happier after quitting because I had more free time. My hair grew back fuller, and my skin and nails looked healthier. Again, this is not the fault of the diet, but rather how challenging it is to eat enough when exercising a lot. I still struggle with the ethics and the treatment of farm animals, so I try to limit the quantity of meat I buy and only support small local farmers (even with vegetables). For the most part, much of my diet is still plant-based, except for cheese, eggs, and honey, and about 50 percent of my meals are raw. I don't drink milk and meat makes less than 5 percent to 10 percent of my diet, sometimes not at all. If I weren't so busy and had time to accurately measure everything, I would do it again in a heartbeat. It is just more work and too challenging to stay on top of your nutrients."

TRUTHS

The raw-food diet is based on the idea that cooking food above about 104 degrees Fahrenheit is harmful. Basically, in the raw-food world, cooking the food essentially "kills" it, removing beneficial nutrients and enzymes, making the food harder to digest, and producing toxins. Foods are eaten raw, fermented, juiced, pureed, or dehydrated to preserve the food's life energy.

Does It Work?

The raw-food diet certainly can contribute to weight loss. In one cross-sectional study of over 500 men and women eating various degrees of raw food (from 70 percent to 100 percent raw) for at least approximately 3.7 years, an average weight loss of almost 22 lb in men and 26.4 pounds in women was seen (71). The higher the percentage of raw foods eaten, the more weight seemed to be lost in this study. Unfortunately, among the women under 45, so much weight was lost that about 30 percent of the group had amenorrhea, and those who ate 90 percent raw or higher had the most women with amenorrhea (71). This is definitely problematic.

A large part of the reason for the extreme weight loss in a raw-food diet is that it tends to consist largely of lower-calorie foods such as raw vegetables. Furthermore, cooked foods appear to provide significantly more calories than raw foods do (72-73). You'd basically have to eat rawer foods to match the caloric intake of a diet that includes cooked foods. Once again, it comes down to creating a caloric deficit.

The Good

The insulin-like growth factor (IGF-1) was lower in the raw-food diet folks in the bone mass study (78). IGF-1 has been connected to certain cancers such as breast cancer and prostate cancer, so this may mean a connection to lowered risk of these types of cancers and a raw-food diet.

The raw foodists in this study also had very low levels of C-reactive protein, which is a marker of inflammation in the body. Chronic inflammation in the body has been linked to the development of a number of diseases, such as diabetes, many types of cancer, hardened arteries, nonalcoholic fatty liver disease, Alzheimer's disease and other types of age-related cognitive impairment, inflammatory bowel disease, and many more (79-80); much of that is related to a deficiency in nutrients such as magnesium, vitamin D, and vitamin K; a low intake of omega-3 fatty acids (either from algae or from fish); a low intake of fruit and veggies; and a high intake of high-glycemic foods like sugar and white flour (81). There are also many lifestyle factors that contribute to chronic low-grade inflammation, such as smoking, high stress levels, insufficient sleep, sedentary lifestyles, and pollution within the environment. Those who consume raw foods most certainly eat way more fruits and veggies than the average person, so that helps a lot. It may also be that raw foodists tend to have more active lifestyles, have less stress, sleep better, and so forth. So it's hard to say exactly why their C-reactive protein markers are so low, but they're clearly doing something right in that regard.

DOWNSIDES

Not only does a raw-food diet contribute to extreme weight loss, but it may also contribute to bone loss. In one study that compared 18 raw foodists eating between 1,285 and 2,432 calories per day to a control group eating a standard American diet containing 1,976 to 3,537 calories per day, intakes of calcium and vitamin D were quite low for the raw foodists. In this study, those on the raw-food diet had much lower bone mass in their total body including the low spine, thigh bones, and hips, compared with those of the same age and sex in the control group (78). In addition, the raw foodists in this study ate low amounts of protein (about 9.1 percent of total calories), which could be problematic for maintaining muscle mass and for athletic performance. While there are very few studies examining bone mass and muscle mass in raw foodists, the data in this study provides some cause for concern.

LIES

The tenets of the raw-food diet are based on misconceptions, or, you know, let's just call them lies. They may not be malicious lies, but the fact is that none of them are true. There is no scientific evidence to demonstrate that a raw-food diet is more nutritious than or advantageous to other diets, and there is actually a lot of evidence to the contrary. So let's just go ahead and debunk everything.

> *There is no scientific evidence to demonstrate that a raw-food diet is more nutritious than or advantageous to other diets, and there is actually a lot of evidence to the contrary.*

Let's check out the science. There aren't a ton of studies that have been done on raw foodists. But of those that exist, here's what has been discovered.

Cancer

A major claim of raw-food diet proponents is that the diet can cure, reverse, or protect the body from cancer. Due to their high vegetable and generally high fat intake (raw-food diets tend to make heavy use of nuts, seeds, avocado, and some oils), raw foodists are able to adequately digest plenty of fat-soluble vitamin A and beta-carotene, which is a good thing (although being on a raw-food diet is certainly not a prerequisite to consuming these nutrients) (74). However, there is currently no evidence to support the cancer claims. Much more research is needed to say what, if any, effects the raw-food diet has on cancer.

Enzymes

One argument made by raw-food proponents is that cooking foods destroys beneficial enzymes inherent in raw foods. The problem with this argument is twofold: (1) The body already makes these enzymes on its own, and (2) the enzymes in raw foods are deactivated in the digestive process anyway (75).

Nutrients and Cooking

Another claim made by proponents of the raw-food diet is that cooking food destroys important nutrients and makes food toxic. This is patently false. As a matter of fact, many of the phytochemicals and nutrients that protect against disease become more available to the body when foods are cooked, which throws a wrench in the idea that a raw-food diet is superior for fighting disease (76-77). Different vegetables seem to have unique reactions to various cooking methods, so depending on the vegetable in question, boiling, steaming, baking, or frying might have different effects on the nutrients of that particular item (76-77). However, many antioxidants and other valuable phytonutrients appear to be best absorbed through cooked food (76-77). Another thing to keep in mind is that cooking food correctly kills a lot of the germs that cause food poisoning. I really don't recommend food poisoning if you can avoid it.

■ Wrap It Up

A raw-food diet has lots of fruits and vegetables, which is great. However, there's no proof that a raw-food diet cures cancer, nor is there any evidence demonstrating that many foods are healthier eaten raw than cooked. Furthermore, there are a lot of foods that are great for you that you simply cannot eat in their raw state (e.g., beans, whole grains, and many protein sources). A raw-food diet also might contribute to extreme weight loss and bone loss as well as nutritional imbalances, so if you want to go this route, be very, very careful.

One more thing: The raw-food diet is a tough one to sustain over time. Making raw-food-type meals can be time-consuming, and unless you mostly socialize with other raw foodists, social events might be difficult when they involve food. Keep all this in mind and plan accordingly if this is a lifestyle that interests you.

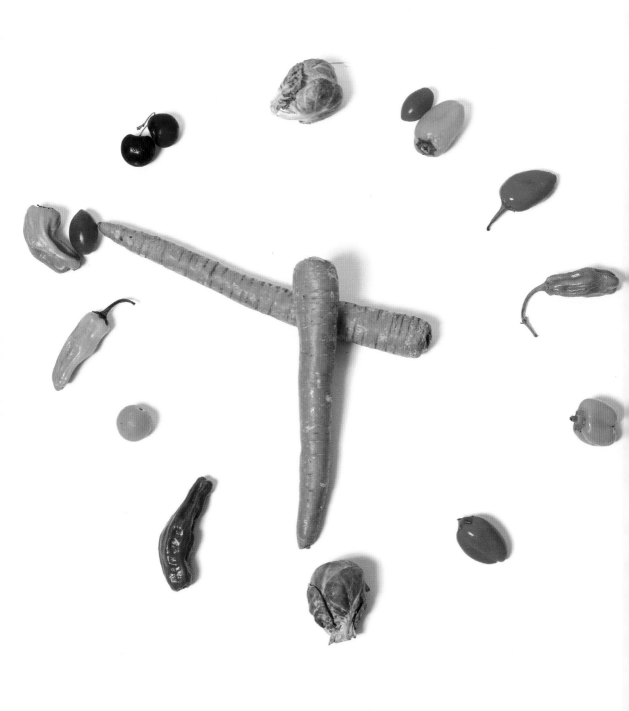

6

Intermittent Fasting

My friend Maksim shared his experience with intermittent fasting (IF):

"I am currently 34 years old, turning 35 in a month. I have been intermittent fasting for roughly the last 10 years and have consistently stayed between 195 and 205 pounds (8-12 percent body fat), and as I write this I am sitting at 203 pounds and 12.2 percent body fat. As with all diets, it's basically an experiment on your body, so you tweak things as needed to accommodate what works for you, so when I say intermittent fasting, it's technically my version of it and not the strict protocol that one may find in literature. Also, I am currently deconditioned and detrained because for the last nine weeks, the state, the country, and most of the world have been under a quarantine lockdown due to a virus pandemic, and I know it's no excuse but I'm owning the fact that I have been a slacker for a bit longer than the nine weeks under quarantine. However, due to my eating regimen and also my work (I'm a trainer and work at a physical therapy clinic so I am on my feet for over eight hours a day), I have been able to keep my body composition and not gain body fat.

Another time that I was able to keep my weight and body fat in check while being sedentary through intermittent fasting was when I ruptured my Achilles tendon three years ago and was not weight bearing or walking for over four months. IF does work and can potentially yield great results, but it is definitely not for everyone and in my opinion should not be done every day. I cycle five days on with two days off on the weekend, where I enjoy fun meals and have more meals throughout the day.

I started IF inadvertently when I was 25 and started working as a personal trainer at 24 Hour Fitness. I had clients starting at 5 a.m. so I would sleep until the last minute, get up, get dressed, make coffee, jet out the door and train clients until about 1 p.m. Then I would have my first meal of the day, which usually was a pretty large meal (2,000-3,000+ calories), and unfortunately it wasn't always the healthiest, especially if I didn't pack a lunch and had to eat out somewhere nearby. Then I would return back to work and train clients (while snacking on nuts, fruits, shakes, etc.) until about 8 p.m. Dinner was usually around 9 p.m. or so and also fairly large, maybe ice cream for dessert, and then sleep. So my fasting window was roughly 15 to 16 hours, depending on how late dinner went on and my first meal the next day. This went on for about five months until I started graduate school and due to an even busier schedule this was the most ideal eating regimen that worked for me. Around 2014, I heard about a book by Ori Hofmekler called *The Warrior Diet*, which outlines intermittent fasting in detail and its history and realized that I have been doing this, or my version of it for a while now! It is now May 2020 and I am still doing IF Monday through Friday with the weekends being a free-for-all because fun meals are very important!"

TRUTHS

IF is basically the practice of going without food, or at least undereating, for a specified period of time on a regular basis. There are a few different ways IF has been structured, including the following:

- *The Warrior diet* is one of the original IF-type diets to become popular. Basically, during a 20-hour period during the day, very little is eaten—maybe some raw fruits and veggies, some hard-boiled eggs, and a little dairy—but that is about it. After the fasting period, you have a four-hour window to have at it. The diet (like many of the IF diets) recommends sticking to whole, unprocessed foods as much as possible.

- *Fasting twice per week* typically involves having 250 to 300 calories per day on fasting days, although some people simply do not consume any calories at all on fasting days; normal eating patterns are resumed for the rest of the week. This format is known as the 5:2 diet. The 5:2 diet is very similar to the *eat-stop-eat* method, which is a version of IF that involves two 24-hour fasting periods once or twice every week, with normal eating resuming all other days. If you eat at 6 p.m. on Monday, for instance, you cannot not eat again until 6 p.m. on Tuesday, thus concluding one 24-hour fast. During fasting, no calories are permitted, although calorie-free beverages are allowed.

- *Alternate-day fasting* is a more extreme version of IF in which fasting occurs every other day, alternating with normal eating days. Some people eat up to 500 calories on fasting days, whereas others choose not to eat at all on fasting days.

- *The 16/8 method* limits eating to about eight hours per day, with fasting taking place the rest of the day. There is some leeway with the fasting hours and eating hours, with some people fasting 14/10, 15/9, 18/6, or some other variation on this theme. This essentially works out to skipping a meal (breakfast or dinner, usually). The eight-ish hours you spend asleep after dinner can help the fasting go a little easier.

- *Unstructured/spontaneous IF* entails skipping meals now and then, whenever desired. For people who don't need a regimented program or whose schedules fluctuate a lot, this may be a more appealing IF option.

Does It Work?

IF is essentially another way to restrict calories. Combining limited time in which food is allowed with general recommendations to eat whole, unprocessed foods reduces opportunities for binging and does not allow for eating as many high-calorie junk foods that are easy to overeat. It can be tough to surpass all the calories you need for the day in one sitting, especially if you're not eating junk foods. I mean, it can be done (I'm pretty sure I've done it every Thanksgiving), but it can be tough. So eating fewer calories just kind of happens when you're following an IF protocol.

While there aren't many studies currently available on the subject, IF in general has been shown to be a successful weight loss strategy in comparison to no strategy at all (82). IF seems to be about as effective (not much more, not much less) than other weight loss methods tested for up to a year (studies to date have not been done for longer than a year) (82). So while it *is* an effective strategy, it is not the best, nor is it the worst strategy out there.

The Good

Many health claims are made about fasting, and there is some evidence to back some of it up. One meta-analysis noted that intermittent fasting, at least up to 12 weeks (no longer IF studies were available at the time this analysis was performed) seemed to preserve muscle better than regular caloric restriction in overweight and obese people (82). However, most of the IF studies analyzed used different (and less reliable) methods of body fat assessment than the majority of the other types of caloric restriction studied, so this may not actually be a valid point.

There is a theory that because food supply in hunter-gatherer times was unpredictable, causing humans and other predatory animals to go long periods of time without eating, the body flips a sort of metabolic switch to keep functioning in top form (84). People and animals who survived and thrived with less food had the advantage and passed those traits on to their offspring.

In animal studies, there seem to be several health benefits associated with IF. When studied in rodents, IF has demonstrated effects ranging from increasing longevity, lowered cancer risk, improved heart rate and blood pressure values, and even seemed to mitigate a lot of the issues associated with a high-fat diet (84). It even improved measures of brain function that tend to go downhill with aging.

> *In the studies that exist, IF lowers body fat comparably to other calorie-restricted diets.*

Research on fasting in humans, however, is much sparser. In the studies that exist, IF lowers body fat comparably to other calorie-restricted diets, as mentioned earlier (82). Several studies indicate that IF improves some risk factors of heart disease (e.g., lowering blood pressure and cholesterol), but this could also be due to the health benefits that come along with fat loss (84). Some studies show that these benefits are more prevalent in IF than in other weight loss methods, but others do not, so there isn't anything conclusive on whether or not IF is superior to anything else for heart health in humans.

LIES

Most of the health benefits attributed to fasting have been demonstrated in rodents. Humans are not rodents and don't process things the same way rodents do, so we can't really draw good conclusions about humans from these studies, even if they are interesting.

While there has been some benefit to IF in cardiovascular disease and diabetes management in humans, the evidence does not indicate that fasting is better than any other caloric-restriction methods for either of these issues. There is very little research on humans for IF, and most of it has been done on obese or overweight subjects in the absence of regular exercise. The heart and blood sugar benefits could be simply the benefits of weight loss, rather than from fasting per se.

There haven't been many studies on IF effects on athletic performance, but there are a handful that have examined the relationship between IF and endurance training, between IF and strength training, and between IF and high-intensity training. Most of these studies have been done on observers of Ramadan, during which the custom is to fast from sunrise to sunset for 28 to 30 days. Even within this population, the results of fasting on weight loss, nutrient consumption, heart disease, diabetes, and other health factors vary greatly depending on the geographic location and customs of the group studied (85). As far as sport performance, fasting does not seem to have any athletic benefit from the studies that currently exist (86).

Wrap It Up

For the most part, IF works about as well as any other caloric-restriction protocol for weight loss. It can be a good way to go for people who don't mind going for long periods without food, provided that they don't overdo it during the eating window. We don't really have much scientific information on normal-weight people or athletes, so there's not much else to say on the subject. There are also no long-term studies to date on IF, so we can't specify any benefits over time. Although there are plenty of anecdotal stories about benefits people have gotten from fasting, science has yet to catch up with the anecdotes. For now, the jury is still out on fasting.

TO OPEN, LIFT TAB.

GLUTEN FREE

ROTINI

Nutrition Facts
6 servings per container
Serving size 2 oz
Amount Per Serving

Calories

Total Fat 1g
Saturated Fat 0g
Trans Fat 0g
Cholesterol 0mg
Sodium 0mg
Total Carbohydrate 44g
Dietary Fiber 2g
Soluble Fiber 1g
Insoluble Fiber 1g
Total Sugars 4g
Protein 7g

Gluten Free™
Delicious White Pasta with 4 Grains

ELBOW

Pasta Your Whole Family
Can Enjoy!

Renned Gluten Free™ pasta
it is produced in a dedicated

Best if Used By
MAY 02 2022
123M051 04:32

To open,
lift tab

Gluten Fr

ELBOW

Gluten Free™
ELBOW

Nutrition Facts
About 6 servings per container
Serving size 1/2 cup (56g)
Amount per serving

Calories 200

% Daily Value*

Total Fat 1.5g   2%
Saturated Fat 0g   0%
Trans Fat 0g
Polyunsaturated Fat 0.5g
Monounsaturated Fat 0.5g

TO OPEN, LIFT TAB.

GLUTEN FREE

Gluten Free™

7

Gluten-Free Diet

My friend Renata and her husband Gary have been on the gluten-free (GF) diet for three years now. This is what Renata had to say about it:

"We were recommended by Gary's doctor to go gluten-free to address some of Gary's health issues. We didn't lose weight, but that wasn't really the goal.

I love how it makes my digestive system feel. For Gary, gluten gives him headaches.

At first, it was hard to find the right substitutes, but now, I can make GF cookies that taste like they aren't GF!

We will always be GF, and I'm dairy-free too.

Every once in a while, if we are in a place that I may not be able to experience a food again, I will eat it, but I pay for it one to three days later with bloating and constipation.

People make GF out to be a bigger deal than it is. My biggest advice is to accept that the food may taste a little different than what you're used to; but give it time and you won't know the difference. Your body will, though."

TRUTHS

One thing I often hear from clients and friends who are trying to lose weight or get healthier is that they have to cut out gluten. When I ask why, they generally say something vague about inflammation and leave it at that. So let's talk a little bit about gluten.

Essentially, gluten is the stuff that makes dough stretchy. It's a kind of protein found in many types of grains. Gluten is an allergen for some people, particularly in cases of wheat allergy, gluten intolerance, and celiac disease. In those people, gluten can cause a whole bunch of not-so-pleasant symptoms, and a gluten-free diet is generally indicated. However, many of the people who are purchasing gluten-free products (a

15.5 billion dollar industry as of 2016, by the way [87]) tend not to have health issues related to gluten at all (88). Are they on the right track?

Does It Work?

Maybe. To date, there is little reliable evidence that gives a proven link between a GF diet and weight loss (89). In one of the only studies done on the subject, people who were following a gluten-free diet had a lower body mass index, higher weight loss, and waist circumference than the general population (89). It is important to note, however, that the data came from self-reported information from surveys and not a controlled, randomized study. This leaves a lot of room for error; the reporting is basically hinging on the assumption that people are being totally honest about all of their information. The fact of the matter is, though, that many people exaggerate (or underestimate) self-reported data, leave important information out, and fudge things for various reasons. It is, unfortunately, not the most reliable data out there, although we can glean at least some information from it.

Another issue with the study is that we cannot say for sure that the GF diet is the reason for the reported fat loss measures, or for any of the other information reported. While it's possible that the GF diet might be useful for weight loss, we simply cannot say for sure. It may be that the people who ate GF foods are simply more health-conscious or more active, or any number of things.

> *A gluten-free diet will certainly limit the foods available to eat, which should create a decrease in calories. However, the GF replacements for the eliminated foods are often not lower in calories than their glutenful counterparts.*

A GF diet will certainly limit the foods available to eat, which should create a decrease in calories. However, the gluten-free replacements for the eliminated foods are often not lower in calories than their gluten-ful counterparts. If you're replacing one food with a food with equal or more calories, you're probably not going to lose weight that way.

The bottom line is that the GF diet might be useful for weight loss, but it's simply not possible to say for sure with the currently available data. Unless it accompanies lowering calories (or unless a GF diet in and of itself somehow burns more calories than a gluten-y diet), it's unlikely that in and of itself a GF diet will be particularly useful for fat loss.

Lies

What about the health claims? Let's break a few of them down.

Gluten Is Inflammatory

Well, yes and no. If you have celiac disease or a gluten allergy, gluten can definitely cause inflammation in your body. However, if you're a healthy human, there's no reliable evidence showing that gluten will increase your inflammation levels.

A Gluten-Free Diet Is Healthier

Once again, I gotta say, "It depends." Does your gluten-free diet accompany lots of fruits and veggies, whole foods, and minimal junk-type foods? Then, yeah, a GF diet is probably healthier for you—but not because of the lack of gluten. On the other hand, a lot of gluten-free foods aren't exactly the most nutritious foods on the market. In fact, GF diets have been linked to a higher risk of cardiovascular disease, potentially *because* they eliminate the consumption of many whole grains (91).

The quality of the available studies on gluten and health varies, but we can glean some information from what we currently know. Gluten consumption does not appear to be linked to a higher risk of heart disease (91), colitis (92), and type 2 diabetes (93). Gluten seems to have a protective effect in men (but not in women) for colorectal cancer, but there may be a potential increased risk of proximal colon cancer (the first half of the colon, closest to the small intestine) related to higher gluten intake for both men and women (94).

A GF diet often becomes nutritionally incomplete, especially when there is a dependence on packaged gluten-free products. GF diets tend to be much lower in fiber as well as a number of vitamins and minerals (95). If you're going to go gluten-free, it's important to pay close attention to the quality of the food you eat. For fiber, it is recommended to eat what is known as *pseudocereals*, which are naturally gluten-free foods that aren't grass-based (cereal grains are grasses) but that you can use like grains (95). Some popular examples of pseudocereals are amaranth, buckwheat, chia, and quinoa. It's also a good idea to make sure you include plenty of veggies and fruits and other whole foods to complete your diet.

It is important to note that most of this research comes from cohort studies, which are observational studies that look at information available about large groups of people and attempt to figure out relationships between that information and diseases. Although cohort studies can provide some useful information, they can't provide a definite cause of a disease. There are also other issues that can skew cohort study data (e.g., there might be missing or inaccurate information, people might drop out of the cohort or pass away, etc.). So while we can get some ideas about the relationship between gluten intake and disease risk, we won't get the whole picture from studies like these. Still, it seems that gluten probably isn't evil, and if you're healthy, you're just fine keeping it in your diet.

■ Wrap It Up

GF diets are imperative if you have celiac disease or a gluten allergy. If you don't, cutting gluten doesn't seem to have any magical weight loss or health-improving effects. Carry on.

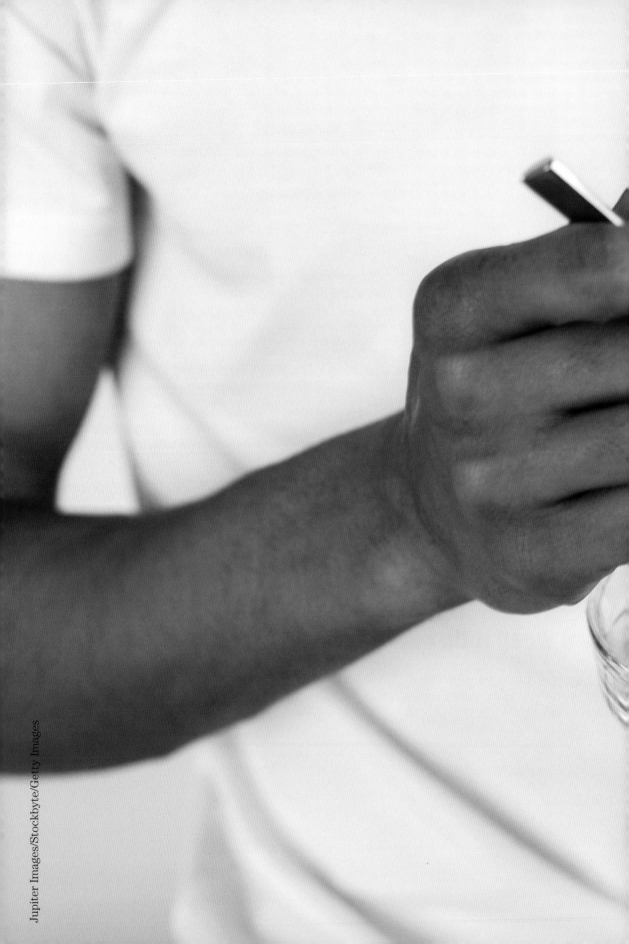

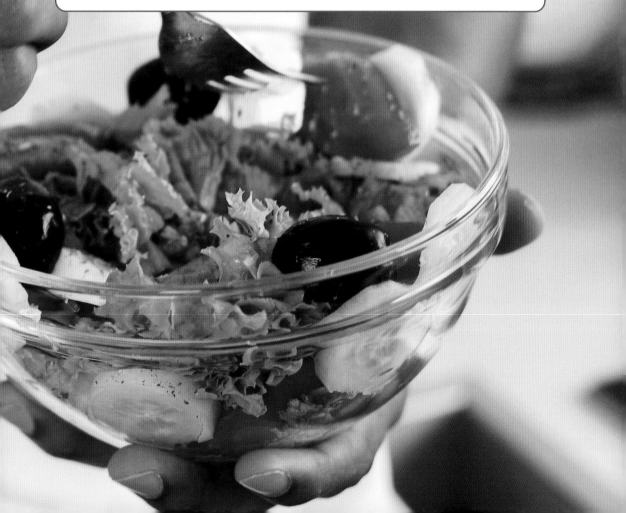

8

Blood Type Diet

My friend Tony explained his experience with the Blood Type diet:

"Back in 2000, between February and December, I gained quite a bit of weight. I had just left a job that was about 90 percent physical labor. I was in the best shape of my life, but I had terrible habits. I could eat and drink whatever I wanted because I'd 'burn it all off' just by doing my job. Once I left that job, my eating and drinking habits remained. But the physical activity was gone. So I gradually put on about 40 pounds over the course of 10 months, hitting the 200-pound mark. I saw an old coworker from that same in December and he jokingly called me 'Gordito' ('Chubby' in Spanish). That's when I realized I had to change my habits.

I went on the Eat Right for Your Blood Type diet by Dr. D'Adamo. The diet basically says that people should eat certain foods based on what people ate in the regions where the different blood types first appeared. For example, type A blood supposedly first appeared when type O people migrated from regions where meat was the primary food source into areas where the primary food sources was more agrarian. This was fascinating to me. But being a carnivore who has type A blood, I was not happy when I realized I had to heavily cut meat from my diet. However, I did see a difference in a rather short amount of time.

I was eating more fish and less beef, more beans and greens, more soy and less dairy, less alcohol . . . So it's no surprise that I was feeling great and back down 30 to 40 pounds in a few months. But I don't think it has anything to do with my blood type. I think it was just a change in my diet and eating habits, combined with healthier food choices. I feel like most diets initially have a good result because you are making conscious choices about what and how much food you put in your mouth. I don't eat as well these days, and my waistline proves it, but I took what I learned and do my best to eat better."

TRUTHS

A fair number of my clients and friends have told me that they can't eat certain foods because their blood type isn't compatible with that dietary road. Are they on to something? Is the Blood Type diet the secret to weight loss and other good stuff?

The Blood Type diet assigns a set of food rules to each blood type in the ABO spectrum; the theory is that certain blood types will thrive under certain dietary conditions and suffer under others. The diet was created by a naturopathic doctor named Peter D'Adamo, who wrote a very popular book on the subject. The basic tenets are as follows:

• *Type A.* According to D'Adamo, people with type A blood have lower stomach acid levels and a specific enzymatic makeup that causes difficulty digesting most animal products and animal fats. They should therefore aim for a more vegetarian diet. Veggies, fish, whole grains, tofu, and turkey are good. Stay away from dairy, wheat, kidney beans, and corn for weight loss. Avoid strenuous exercise; stick to low-impact workouts like tai chi, walking, yoga, and Pilates.

• *Type B.* A person with blood type B can allegedly eat the whole spectrum of foods healthfully. However, certain types of meat and seafood should be avoided due to there being a higher risk of stroke and other issues for type B'ers. Dr. D'Adamo claims that many types of wheat in the type B system will affect metabolism negatively, may increase risk of some diseases, or will simply not be well digested. Medium- to rare-cooked goat, lamb, and mutton are preferred meat sources as well as fatty cold-water fish. Avoid chicken, peanuts, corn, and wheat when trying to lose weight. Low-fat items are problematic. Exercise can be low-impact to moderate, including hiking, swimming, martial arts, bicycling; and tai chi, yoga, and Pilates.

• *Type AB.* Blood type AB, according to D'Adamo, inherits some of the dietary needs of type A and type B. An AB-type person, like type A, has lower stomach acid levels, making many animal products difficult to digest. The AB type will also have difficulty digesting certain combinations of foods, so they should, for instance, eat protein and starch separately. AB type folks should steer clear of red meat; soy and fatty cold-water fish should be the main protein sources. Yogurt and other cultured dairy products are OK, but uncultured dairy, such as fresh milk, can cause digestive issues or increase disease risk. Avoid wheat,

SOMETHING TO KEEP IN MIND

A diet book automatically gets more credence in the eyes of many consumers if the author is a doctor. As the daughter of two doctors, I can tell you with great confidence that doctors are not always the best sources of nutritional information. Thorough studies in nutrition are not generally part of a medical curriculum, and unless your doctor has had considerable education in the nutrition field, that author may not be the best authority on the subject. If you're choosing a diet simply because it was doctor-created or recommended, be sure that you understand the doctor's background first.

chicken, corn, buckwheat, and kidney beans. Exercise can be low-impact to moderate, including hiking, swimming, martial arts, bicycling; and tai chi, yoga, and Pilates.

• Type O. Dr. D'Adamo purports that type O blood corresponds to higher levels of stomach acid, meaning most types of meat can be digested well, and apparently the combination of protein and fat digests particularly well for type O'ers. At the same time, type O people convert grains to triglycerides and fat, causing a negative immune response. This type cannot be vegetarian healthfully and basically is recommended a Paleo-type diet. Eat lots of animal protein, veggies, fruit, and fish. Stay away from beans and grains (like the low-carbohydrate diets). Avoid corn, wheat, and dairy products for weight loss. Type O digests fat well, so low-fat items are not digested well. Perform vigorous aerobic exercise for up to an hour per day.

Does It Work?

The Blood Type diet gives some decent advice. It's based on whole foods and tends to recommend lots of veggies and fish and, in some cases, beans and whole grains. If you're following the Blood Type diet, chances are you're also cutting out a bunch of not-so-good-for-you foods and drinks, which generally means better health and fewer calories (and fewer calories tends to translate to fat loss).

The various dietary recommendations are restrictive, though, and can be hard to stick to for many. Furthermore, cutting specific foods out of the diet such as whole grains or legumes could be unnecessarily removing some healthy foods out of your diet. And there is absolutely no reason, regarding blood type, to cut any of those foods out of your diet.

> *The thing is that none of these positive results in these studies were linked to blood type.*

LIES

There is very little research on the Blood Type diet. One study concluded that there is absolutely no evidence linking blood type to health effects of diet (96). Another study showed that there are, in fact, some health benefits to following different aspects of the Blood Type diet (97). Following the AB diet, for instance, resulted in better blood pressure, cholesterol, triglycerides, insulin, and other favorable health factors. Following the A diet demonstrated all these results, as well as a lower body mass index and waist circumference. Following the type O diet resulted in lower triglycerides. A third study also showed some benefits to following certain tenets of the Blood Type diet—type A diets tended to have lower blood pressure, type B and type AB diets tended to have lower waist circumference, and type O diets had lower body mass index and waist circumference (98). The thing is that none of the results in these studies were linked to blood type. In other words, someone with type O blood could follow the type A diet and get healthier. The link between blood type and diet is simply not there.

Wrap It Up

The Blood Type diet might help you lose weight if it results in cutting calories and might give some other health benefits, but it's got nothing to do with blood type.

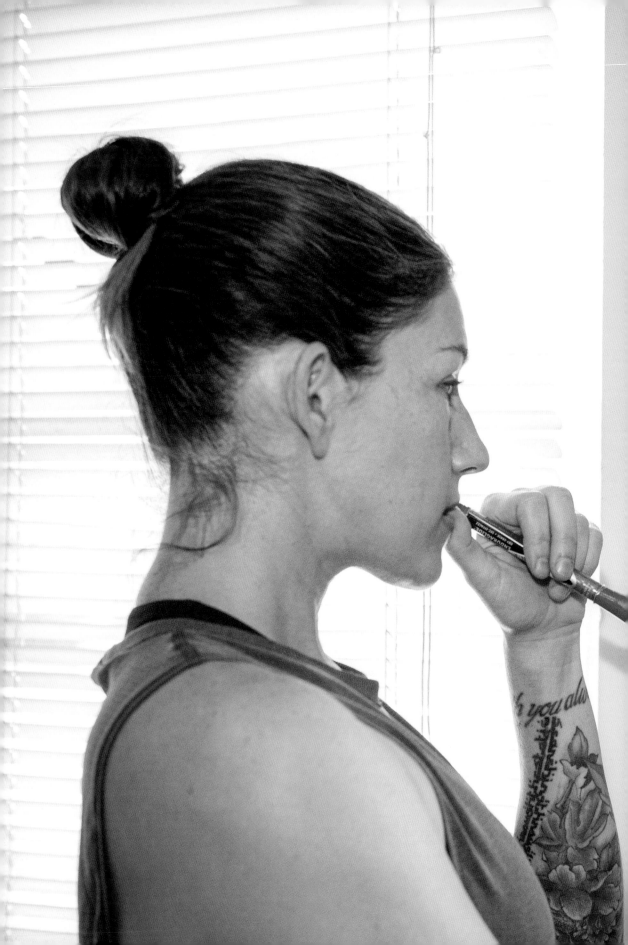

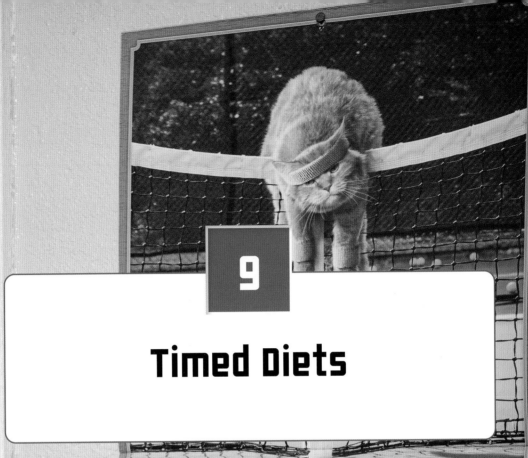

9

Timed Diets

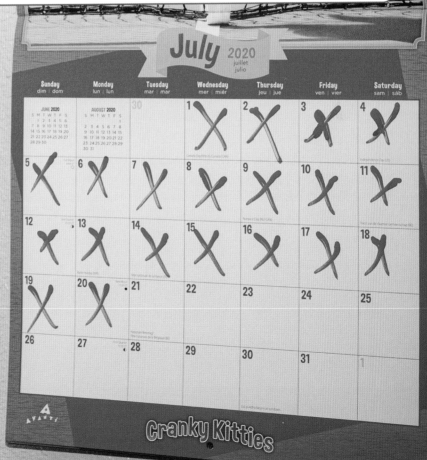

My friend Pete told me about his experience on a six-week, 20-pound weight loss program at a local gym chain:

"I've been heavy my whole life and I've worked out occasionally but never really exerted myself at the gym so when I saw social media ads for a six-week program, I decided to try. I had a friend who did it with good results and they promised to support and help me. I was promised it would be free as long as I lost the required 20 pounds in six weeks.

I hated it. It was way too hard, and I wanted to quit after every session. But along the way I met some great people and I stuck it out for them, and we started a little workout group. Progress was slow but steady and my weight fluctuated for the first few weeks. But I (mostly) stuck to the food plan and did the daily workouts. As the sixth week approached, I was behind schedule, so I followed their program for that and had to eat only tilapia and asparagus for each meal. I honestly didn't think I could do it. But on the final weigh in, I ended up losing 20.6 pounds.

Since the program was free, I decided to repeat the process. I lost another 20 pounds. But toward the end I injured my knee and shoulder. I had to go to physical therapy and slacked off on the program. My injuries never fully recovered, and I spoke with a nutritionist, who told me that this type of program was unsustainable and that there were other ways. I ended up just going back to my old habits and have gained most of that weight back. But overall, I liked the program. The friendships that I made still exist and I was proud of myself for completing the six-week program twice and I admit I looked and felt better."

My friend Nelida also shared her experience with a timed diet: "I joined the program because it looked slightly different than all the other diets I'd tried in the past (without success), and seemed relatively easy to use. No counting or weighing or measuring! I paid my money (which they said they would refund after the initial three months if I lost weight), downloaded the app, weighed and measured myself, took selfies from all the angles, and then set about my life.

For three months I followed their eating plan, using their app, weighing myself weekly, and taking weekly photos. I could see and feel my weight dropping, and it was working. It was a very easy program to follow, and the app was really user friendly. I joined the Facebook group and saw others doing the same things I was doing, and they were also having success.

Then the same thing happened, which always happens when I'm on a diet—I lost interest at about month 2 because it became boring to log, photograph, weigh, and measure myself weekly. Also, some personal stuff was happening, and I reverted to my usual coping mechanisms of eating as much food as possible to dull the emotions I was feeling. However, I kept going just so I could get my money back. The reality is that I was lying in my recording of the foods I was eating, and I stopped taking photos and weighing and measuring myself. I put all the weight that I'd lost back on, with some extra for good measure. In the end, they didn't give me my money back because I hadn't read the small print properly and hadn't followed the extremely strict instructions they had for refunds."

TRUTHS

Timed diets are a basic category that I am using to describe diets that have a set amount of time you're supposed to be on them; for instance, a "six-week challenge" at a gym or at work, or something along those lines. These types of diets often have a goal of rapid weight loss and some provide a reward if you hit a specific weight loss poundage (e.g., a gym in my neighborhood offers a money-back guarantee if you lose 20 lb within six weeks on their program).

Does It Work?

There are a lot of different kinds of timed diets, and most of them involve a pretty restrictive eating pattern. In most cases, this means you will be eating fewer calories and will likely lose weight as a result.

LIES

There are a few issues with these diets, although they aren't lies per se. First, virtually none of these very restrictive diets are sustainable in the long term. Then again, the programs generally do not promise long-term results—only that you will lose a specific amount of weight. That is generally the attraction. People love the idea of losing weight but don't consider how they'll maintain it going forward.

Most people do not find highly restrictive diets to be satisfying, and there's a good chance that you'll be pretty miserable while you're going through the plan. Second, highly restrictive diets may not provide the nutrition or energy needed in daily life, particularly if intense workouts are also included. While a caloric deficit is important for fat loss, too much of a caloric deficit comes with its own issues. A third issue is that very few of these short-term diets teach people how to eat sustainably long-term. In other words, once you go off the diet, you tend to go back to your old eating patterns (or worse, since you've been deprived for a while), and the weight will likely come back.

Most people do not find highly restrictive diets to be satisfying, and there's a good chance you'll be pretty miserable while you're going through the plan.

While yo-yo dieting will not necessarily mean that you will be at risk for a higher weight gain or diabetes (99), it is certainly not ideal. Losing weight in the short term can be super satisfying. You'll see your weight plummet (particularly at the beginning, mostly due to water loss more than fat loss, although there will likely also be some fat loss), and that feels awesome. Your clothes will fit better, and you might be ready for an event that you were preparing for.

However, when you go off the diet and return to status quo, there's a distinct possibility you might feel depressed, frustrated, or like a failure. Of course, you might not feel any of these things, but they are not uncommon responses to regaining lost weight. That said, there is very little research on the psychological effects of not reaching dieting goals, so I can only go by my own observations.

A very unfortunate fact is that most people who lose even a small percentage (5 to 10 percent) of their body weight gain it back within a year (100). If you want to lose weight and keep it off, finding something you can stick to long-term is important.

■ Wrap It Up

Short-term diets usually work—for the short term. They may not be nutritionally or calorically sound, though, and chances are that most people won't stick to them beyond the prescribed length of the diet. If you want something long-term, look elsewhere.

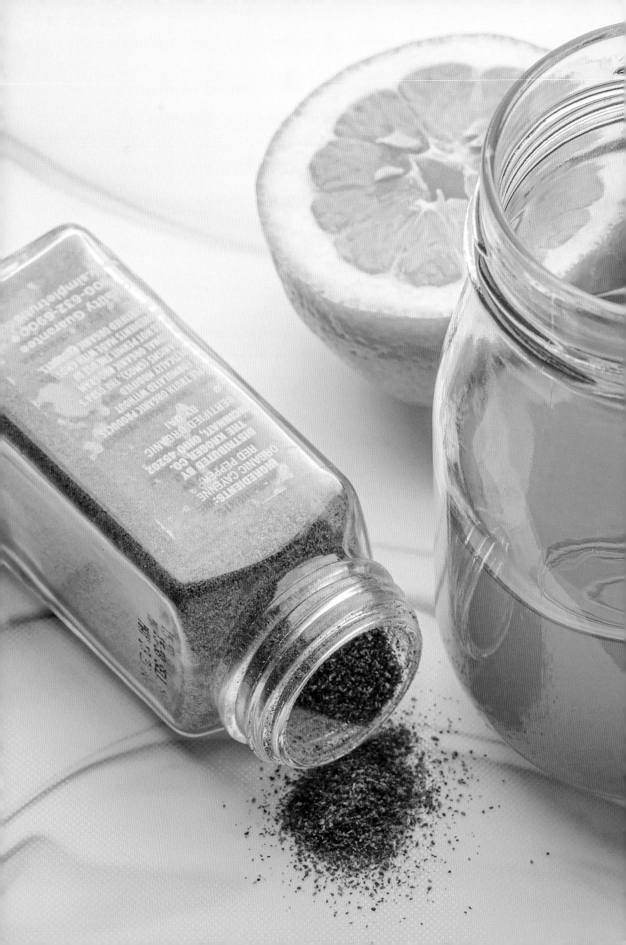

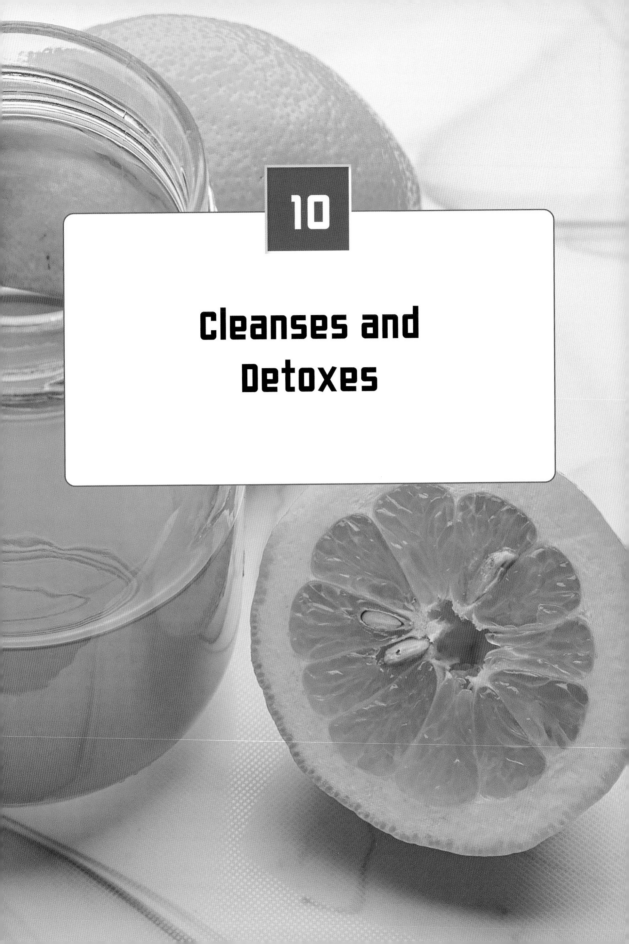

10

Cleanses and Detoxes

Several of my friends offered up their experiences with cleanses.

My friend Corey kept it short and sweet: "I did one a few years ago for a month. I did it, lost a lot of weight, and then I put it back on when I stopped. And I took a lot of supplements. The end."

My friend Philippe had much more to say:

"I experimented with the Master Cleanse back in early 2006. The reasons for it were simple: A friend of mine told me about it, he and his wife had tried it, and while I didn't have an inherent need for it, my nutrition knowledge was more empirical than educational, other than whatever was covered in courses for my personal training accreditation (as in what was covered in the National Academy of Sports Medicine book, as well as a course I took called 'nutrition for athletes').

Mostly in those days, I'd hear or read something, and I would try it on myself so I could talk about it.

I have never suffered any major weight issues other than being a natural ectomorph, skinny teenager, and I would at times put on body fat when eating more to 'gain,' without any precision other than eat more, lift more, and get bigger.

So, when the idea of speeding up my metabolism, getting ready for a photo shoot and jumping on the Master Cleanse bandwagon came up, I said, 'Sure, why not?'

I wanted to see if I could last with discipline and set out a goal of doing it for 10 days.

I started with the non-iodized sea saltwater flush. Did it a few times in the entire period.

Didn't leave the house after doing it. Allegedly, its pH is akin to blood, your body will reject it, and you make frequent trips to the toilet. Having done it two, maybe three, times, I noticed how much 'clearer' any expelled matter was. Grossness alert: The first flush was the big one, more 'colored' and thicker. Subsequent ones were more watery, with some residual food matter (things less digestible, leafy) on the second, and nearly nothing on the third.

I was concerned with the lack of protein, as all I was ingesting was either water or the 'lemonade,' which consisted of water, lemon juice, grade B (dark amber) maple syrup, and cayenne pepper. The warning was that for folks who needed to 'detox' badly, it could cause anxiety, negative emotions, and physical setbacks. While being a relatively sensible eater, I experienced no physical reactions. (I had a client try—a super-fit genetic [anomaly] with a year-round six-pack who ate lots of junk, and she had to stop. She didn't do well.)

Day 1 was OK and exciting. Days 2 to 4 were hunger pangs, shrinking stomach, and borborygmus galore. But I was able to rationalize, 'my stomach wants stuff in it, but I don't need food, I am not hungry, I am still getting enough calories.' Never a dip in energy. Some irritability or food envy (smelling other people's foods was a torture).

The Master Cleanse protocol suggests for people with poor eating habits to drink peppermint tea because the chlorophyll would help with neutralizing the nasty sweat the detox could produce. Like getting gunk out of your system. I experienced no such thing but enjoyed the tea nevertheless for boredom relief from the lemonade–maple syrup–cayenne pepper concoction.

I noticed that my sweat was actually smelling like maple syrup, so it was not unpleasant. My sense of smell was also very sharp, and I had dropped from 183 to 185 pounds to 172 to 173 pounds in that 10-day period. I never felt weak, it was easy to get through the day by staying busy and always having a jug of 'juice' by my side any time I felt hungry. Senses alert: I even went to a BBQ the day before the end of my cleanse and remained disciplined with the plan.

I ended my fast with a chocolate croissant and orange juice (not a soup or broth as recommended) and felt fine, no gastrointestinal issues or others.

I felt my metabolism was accelerated for a while, and it was hard to put on the weight back on. My thought is that my weight loss was part water weight, part fat as well, and mainly all the gunk in my system. I didn't need to go number 2 after day 5 or 6 at all, but I peed a lot (from drinking a lot).

Would I suggest it? Would I do it again? No and no. No, because I don't believe in cleanses; I believe in sensible eating. I am also not a certified nutrition coach. I wouldn't do it because it's off my bucket list, and I fear at my age (46) that losing muscle mass makes it harder to regain.

Did I benefit from it? I think I did, then. I had a few clients do it; they all but one enjoyed the process, and here and there afterward, some would do a flush, a clean-out of their inner gutters, or a two-day version of it (why is up to them). I dug the faster metabolism and ate junk without guilt, remorse or even consequences for what seemed like months following the experience."

TRUTHS

The world of detoxing is extremely alluring. Detoxing claims to purge your body of the toxins it apparently accumulates from everything from diet to air to water to life in general. It can make your skin glow, make your hair gleam, make your teeth and nails strong, make your organs function better, improve your energy levels, reverse diseases, help you think better, help you digest your food better, or make the pounds simply melt off. Is there any truth to the hype?

Most detox diets eliminate specific foods from the diet. This often includes any number of meats, sugars, salts, oils, processed foods, caffeine, soy, certain fruits or vegetables, legumes, wheats, and so on. It may involve fasting, drinking various juice concoctions, sipping on soup or broth, taking laxatives and diuretics, taking probiotics, using sweat therapy (like saunas), or taking various supplements. They may even include enemas or colonics. There may be certain foods recommended as particularly cleansing. A detox may last for only a few days or for longer periods of time.

Does It Work?

Inasmuch as detox diets generally cause an extreme reduction in calories, they can lead to some short-term weight loss. They are almost guaranteed to not be sustainable in the long term, however, which means the weight will likely come back when normal eating patterns resume. Furthermore, very low-calorie diets and highly restrictive diets are generally nutritionally incomplete. If you are deficient in key nutrients long enough, some pretty major health problems can follow, including death (101).

Detox diets can also be very cost prohibitive. A quick Internet search showed me a "superfood detox bundle" for $140, some sort of soup detox for $250, a 3-day juice cleanse for $100, a 5-day "beginner" juice cleanse for $120, a 14-day "detox cleanse" for $176, and a 21-day "cleanse" for $475. There are also endless books on the subject, all of them preaching different formulas for the detox diet du jour. There is no consistency, no regulation, and no scientific proof of any of these diets. But they can be phenomenal moneymakers for their creators.

I get why people are attracted to detoxing. They feel like a fresh start, and their lofty claims are alluring. In many cases, the word *detox* is replaced by other terms like *cleanse* and *renewal*, which make things sound really enticing (and also make them much trickier to regulate). The faces of the detox plans often look calm, confident, at peace, and radiant. It seems like a great way to kick off a brand-new, healthy lifestyle (which, for most, doesn't seem to follow for very long). But in the end, they're simply unproven, murky promises that, in the end, won't be kept.

LIES

The thing about the term *toxins* is that it's not particularly well defined. Street drugs, many medications, alcohol, and tobacco can create addictive patterns and put some pretty poisonous stuff in the body. The process of stopping dangerous addictions is certainly a detoxification process of sorts. But it isn't what these diets are geared toward. Detox diets generally have a very vague definition of what toxins, exactly, they are removing—heavy metals, chemicals in food and drink, pollutants in the air, or perhaps pollutants we absorb through our skin through personal hygiene practices, through our clothing, and anything else we contact during the day. When the term *toxin* is so loosely defined, it becomes pretty hard to prove whether or not it is been effectively removed (or whether it even needs to be), unfortunately (101). And the fact is that the type of toxin we're addressing is important, as is how much of that toxin is in the system. Our bodies are extremely adaptable and can handle small amounts of many "evil" chemicals with no ill effects (101).

> *Detox diets generally have a very vague definition of what toxins, exactly, they are removing . . . .*

That isn't to say that there aren't plenty of chemicals that aren't potentially harmful. Many chemicals previously used in agriculture, packaging, and even in homes (asbestos and lead pipes, anyone?) are banned in many countries due to being linked to various health problems. While there are some animal studies that demonstrate the potential for some food ingredients—such as coriander, chlorella, and citric acid (among a few others)—to remove certain heavy metals and a few other poisonous chemicals from the body, the vast majority of those results have not been proven in humans to date (101). What's more, there certainly has not been any diet that has been shown to remove these or other harmful substances from the body.

Wrap It Up

Detox diets may lead to temporary weight loss. However, they're usually unsustainable, highly restrictive, expensive, and potentially dangerous. There is no science showing benefits to detox diets (101). If you decide to go this route, proceed with caution, and don't get your hopes up too high.

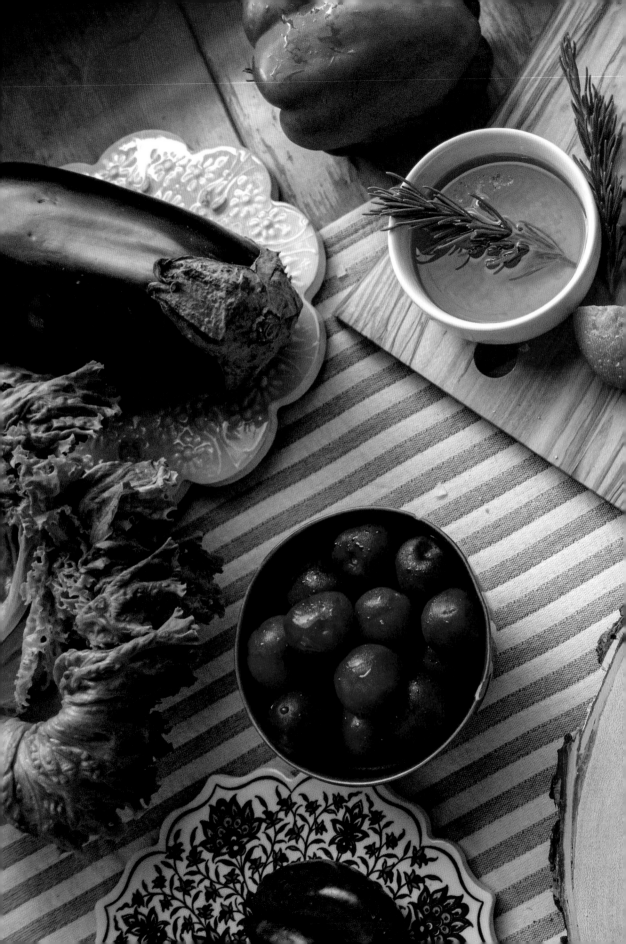

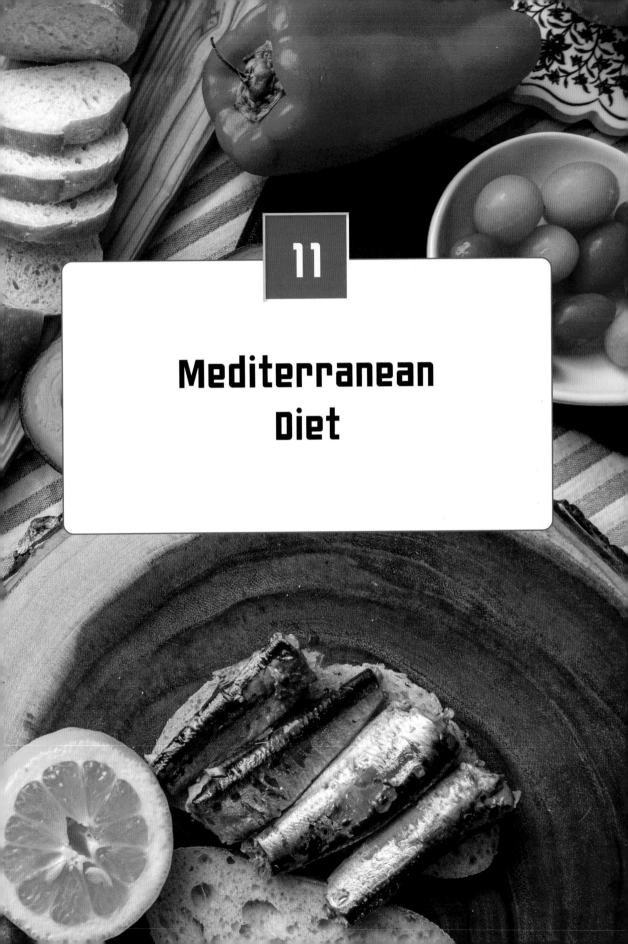

11

Mediterranean Diet

My friend Monique shared with me her experience on the Mediterranean diet:

"I grew up with an old-world Sicilian father. The transition to a 'Mediterranean' diet took absolutely no intentional effort on my part other than journaling and reflecting on how closely my childhood eating habits resembled what was now being promoted as a packaged and intentional diet for those looking to change their eating habits.

Dad didn't like snacking before dinner, so he always set out a relish tray with olives (green and black, cucumbers, tomato wedges, and green onions).

Dinner regularly consisted of some sort of protein—usually fish, lamb, chicken, or pork. Red meat was rare unless Dad was cooking outdoors on the BBQ. Dark-green vegetables and salad were a daily side to any entrée and the usuals were Brussels sprouts, spinach, zucchini, green beans, turnip greens with pearl onions, and salads with romaine because they were 'better for you.'

The only thing that Dad wasn't a stickler about was olive oil. I quickly learned through nutritional studies that this was the way to go with the monounsaturated fat that olive oil provided. No canola, no sunflower, no vegetable oil—just olive oil. I even use it in my baked goods because I just love how it tastes and my kids never notice the difference. I raised them on olive oil with everything. And garlic—if garlic were appropriate in a chocolate chip cookie, I'd probably go there. But I have to draw the line somewhere for the sake of the kids.

The Mediterranean diet that I follow is filled with vegetables, nuts, legumes, seafood, olives, feta, and a variety of other cheeses (within limits), in addition to some of the protein sources I mentioned.

The Hispanic side of my family has influenced me to add some things to the diet that take away from the purity of a Mediterranean-only existence. I am a huge fan of peppers: jalapeño, Anaheim, Ortega, habanero, and the non-spicy relatives—red, orange, yellow, and green bell peppers—all of which are my favorite forms of vitamin C- or metabolism-boosting qualities.

Overall, the primarily Mediterranean diet that I was raised on has afforded me a ton of benefits. My blood pressure has been a steady 100/70 to 110/75. My cholesterol is low. When I have had periods of weight gain due to pregnancy or (more recently) hormonal issues with the onset of menopause, the range is minimal and I honestly believe that I have never had severe symptoms during my menstrual cycle or with menopause. PMS has never been an issue and I've yet to feel what a real hot flash feels like. Honestly, given my history, I don't think it will be what most women say it is because my nutrition is good and my metabolism and muscle-fat ratio works in my favor as a reward for all of the years in the gym.

When I deviate from the Mediterranean diet, I instantly feel a difference in the amount of inflammation in my joints and general achiness that comes with entering the second half of the century. When I am loyal to my eating habits, my achy joints don't bother me, and my energy is amazing.

More recently, I have found that I am more attracted to the idea of eliminating animal products entirely. This will be a process for me, but I feel that it is a necessary one because our meat sources are more and more questionable all the time. Added hormones and questionable practices during production are causing me to reflect and rethink my current protein habits. I just need to find some food combinations that will keep my protein up the way that animal protein has all of these years. I also need to consider my family who is not necessarily on the same page with me regarding living a plant-based existence.

So my next step is to take the Mediterranean diet one step further and refine it to a plant-based Mediterranean diet that is satisfying and nutritionally sound."

TRUTHS

The Mediterranean diet essentially describes the general diet of the people who live in the countries surrounding the Mediterranean Sea. Although the diet doesn't have one concrete definition, it's generally high in veggies, fruits, whole grains, legumes, herbs and spices, fish, and olive oils. Poultry, eggs, and dairy are included more sparingly, and red meat is included only occasionally. Refined meats, sugary meats, and commercially processed meats and snacks are generally avoided in this diet.

Does It Work?

While research specifically studying the Mediterranean diet and weight loss is scarce, the studies that exist show that the diet can work for weight loss. One meta-analysis of five randomized, controlled studies found the Mediterranean diet to be more effective than low-fat diets but about as effective as the low-carb diet and the American Diabetes Association diet for weight loss in obese individuals practicing the diets for more than one year (102). Two more analyses concluded that the Mediterranean diet was better than a control diet for weight loss and did not tend to cause weight gain (103-105). It should be noted that when a Mediterranean diet also included more physical activity or was reduced in calories, it was more effective for weight loss than a standard Mediterranean diet (104-105).

> *Chances are that the Mediterranean diet is useful for weight loss because it doesn't generally include foods we tend to overeat, like snack foods and sweets, and increases foods that keep us fuller for longer.*

The Mediterranean diet has mainly been studied for its health benefits rather than for its effects on weight loss. It has been strongly correlated with a reduction in the risk of cardiovascular disease (102-105). This diet is rich in polyphenols, which are healthful compounds in different plant foods that are full of antioxidants. Olive oil, veggies, fruits, beans, wines, and whole grains are all great sources of polyphenols that are included in the Mediterranean diet. Polyphenols are thought to be behind all kinds of good stuff—protecting the body from disease and degeneration, lowering inflammation, improving gut health and digestion, and more (105). It has been suggested that eating a high-polyphenol diet low in processed foods (like the Mediterranean diet) helps lower inflammation levels and therefore helps lower markers of obesity and metabolic disease (106). While there is research demonstrating that polyphenols play a role in reducing inflammation, act as prebiotics, help burn brown fat tissue, increase satiety (and therefore decrease the desire to eat more), and more, the evidence that polyphenols alone are responsible for weight loss is weak at best (105).

Chances are, the Mediterranean diet is useful for weight loss because it doesn't generally include foods we tend to overeat, like snack foods and sweets, and increases foods that keep us fuller for longer. Because of this, people who embark on a Mediterranean diet likely eat fewer calories than they ate before. When caloric restriction and exercise are added to the Mediterranean diet, fat loss benefits are even better (104-105).

LIES

It also stands to reason that if you're on the Mediterranean diet but are still taking in more calories than you're burning off, you won't see the weight loss benefits from the program and will more than likely gain weight. Because the diet itself isn't super restrictive, it's open to interpretation. While this may be an attractive feature to many, it may also be a problem for those who have issues with portion control. Eating large quantities of oil—even olive oil—and fatty foods like nuts can lead to a high-calorie diet, and that can lead to problems. Even on a diet that is full of super-healthy foods, you still need to watch your portion sizes.

Wrap It Up

The Mediterranean diet can be a healthy way to lose weight if you're keeping your calories in check. Remember—just because a diet is healthy doesn't mean it'll automatically lead to weight loss.

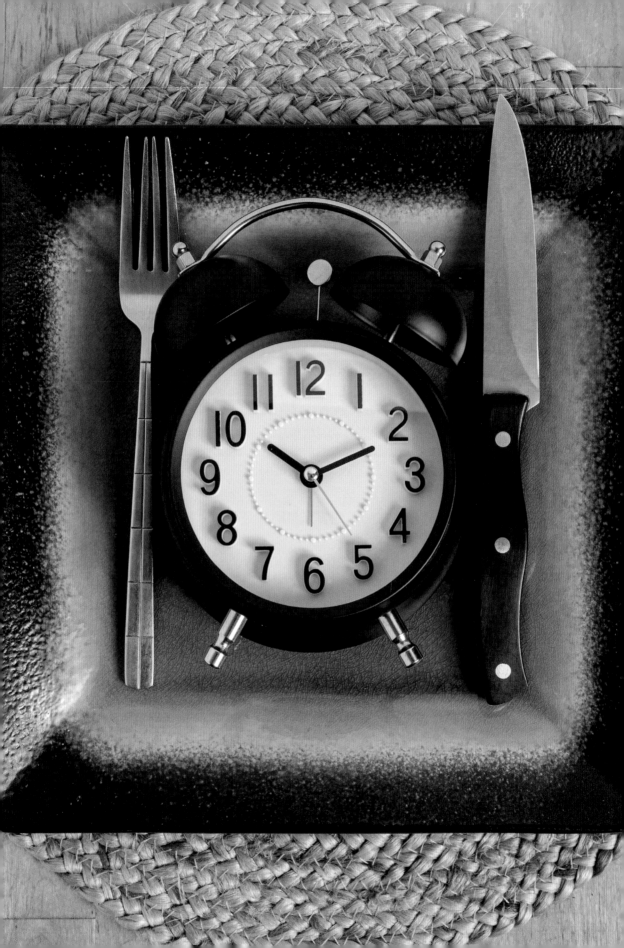

12

Three-Hour Diet

My friend Jeremy shared his experience with eating several small meals per day:

"Ever since about the sixth grade I've always been a little heavy. As I reached adulthood and started raising a family, working long hours, and not focusing on my health, I've gained and lost weight numerous times. What I've finally found that works for me is a consistent approach to nutrition wherein I eat four or five smaller meals per day—not the traditional breakfast, lunch, and dinner. What this has done for me is immense. I've been more successful following this style of nutrition plan than anything else. Eating smaller meals multiple times a day allows me to not feel hungry, and therefore I have greater success in sticking to a good plan and a proper balanced nutrition. It keeps my metabolism burning, constantly putting small piles of wood on a fire to keep it going instead of throwing one giant log on a couple of times a day, which also helps me burn fat and build muscle more consistently. I feel more energetic and I never have any dips in my mental focus or energy. But here's the thing—eating smaller portions multiple times a day isn't a magic bullet. It must be consistent, proper, balanced nutrition. I eat five to six servings of both veggies and lean proteins; three servings of fruit; four servings of starches (I don't say 'carbs,' because technically speaking, fruits and vegetables are also carbs) like potatoes and other root vegetables, whole-grain bread, and brown rice; and some healthy fats like cheese, avocado, nuts, hummus, and heart-healthy oils. As I've gotten older, I've learned that when it comes to weight management and weight loss, lean muscle building, balanced energy, and overall health, I cannot out-exercise a bad diet. It all comes down to consistency, portion control, eating balanced nutrients, and keeping my metabolism revved up by eating smaller portions multiple times a day."

My friend Alison also shared her experience:
"The pros:

1. If I want to attain and maintain a certain bodyweight (for me, that's 132ish pounds), I have to eat that way;
2. My energy is better—I assume it's because my blood sugar is more stable;
3. My athletic performance is better which means my cardio fitness and strength training are all improved.

Cons:

1. Tons of prep time;
2. Carrying food with me everywhere because I'm running so light on fuel;
3. I feel like I'm constantly eating;
4. Life can easily disrupt all of this.

The *only* times I've been able to pull off significant weight loss (I'm talking 30 pounds) are by eating this way, and I have to maintain this habit to maintain the fat loss. Intermittent fasting absolutely does not work for me. Keto tastes great but doesn't help me feel satiated, lose weight, and definitely interferes with my workouts. I'm not currently doing the five to six small meals but I'm just about to get back on the wagon! Whenever I fail to maintain this eating style, I can gain weight quickly—I mean, like, 10 pounds, in the blink of an eye. I think this works best for me because I get reactive hypoglycemia. I have to tend toward low-carb to maintain my blood sugar levels, so my macro breakdown is 40 protein / 30 fat / 30 carbs."

TRUTHS

A popular diet tip that's been around for a while is the idea that eating every three hours or so, or five to six small meals per day, stokes the metabolism, whereas going for a longer time without eating throws the body into a fat-saving starvation mode. This is kind of the opposite idea of fasting—true to form, the world of nutrition is full of contradicting ideas. This idea gained more popularity in 2005 in a book called *The 3-Hour Diet* by Jorge Cruise. The diet touts five smaller, balanced meals spaced at three-hour intervals throughout the day.

Does It Work?

One of the tenets of the three-hour diet is that main meals will hover around 400 calories, and any form of snacking should stay around 100 calories. By the end of the day, you've eaten about 1,400 to 1,500 calories, and for a lot of people, this will lead to weight loss, as many people burn more than 1,500 calories per day (and as it is likely a lot fewer calories than they were consuming before going on this particular diet plan). In fact, for someone who is exercising intensely on a regular basis, this calorie recommendation might be pretty low.

The Good

The three-hour diet doesn't place major restrictions on the types of food people eat, as long as they remain within specific portion sizes for carbohydrates, proteins, and fats. Portion control is absolutely necessary for fat loss, so in this respect, this is a good idea.

The three-hour diet doesn't label foods as "good" or "bad" and doesn't place many limitations on what people can eat. It allows for dietary restrictions (religious, allergen-related, etc.) where needed and has plenty of flexibility for food preferences. This all bodes well for the ability to stick to the diet over time.

The three-hour diet doesn't label foods as "good" or "bad" and doesn't place many limitations on what people can eat.

LIES

The diet works because of caloric restrictions and portion control—not because eating every three hours "stokes your metabolism" (there is very little scientific evidence for this [108]). Furthermore, there isn't any evidence that eating every three hours lowers stress and cortisol levels, as the book claims it does. There is some evidence that eating several small meals a day may keep people feeling less hungry throughout the day (109). This can help stop the likelihood of bingeing that often results from more restrictive diets. However, the research isn't consistent on this—there are also studies that don't show that eating more often leads to less hunger (109). So really, it most likely comes down to personal preference.

Wrap It Up

The three-hour diet, or any form of diet in which you eat several small meals per day, works for weight loss as long as the calories you consume are fewer than the calories you burn off. It has nothing to do with three hours being a magical fat loss number.

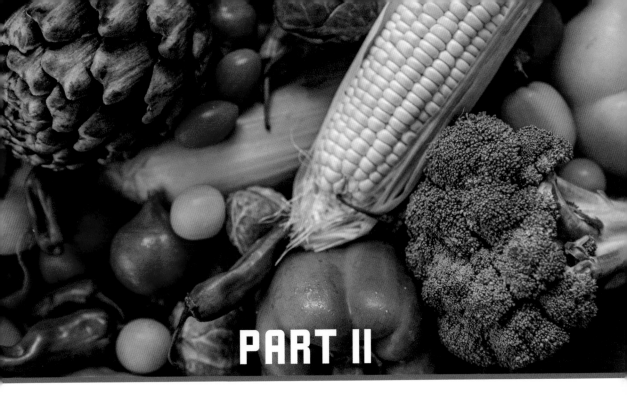

PART II

We've discussed a lot of diet myths and facts, but there's a lot more murkiness in the world of nutrition and fat loss. In the following section, I'm going to talk about a lot of other concepts that often get thrown around regarding food. These are ideas that people commonly accept without actually questioning. I'm a big fan of questioning all the things, though, so perhaps you'll get some food for thought (see what I did there?) about some views you've held dear for a while.

After that, we're going to finally get down to the nitty-gritty—what *is* the best diet, then? What is the magic fat-loss bullet we've all been searching for? Well, stay tuned, and I'll do my best to tell you all that science and experience have told me to date.

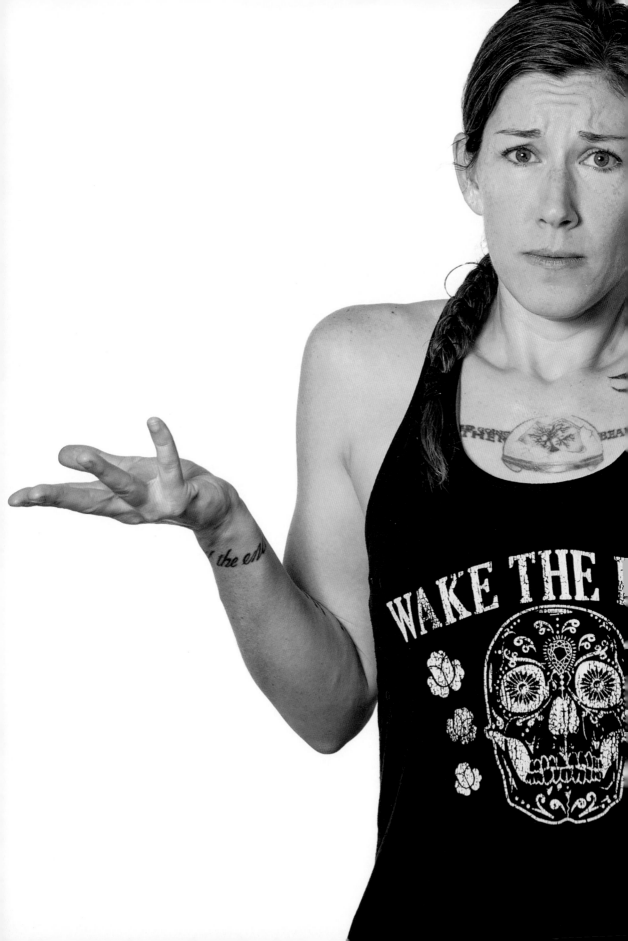

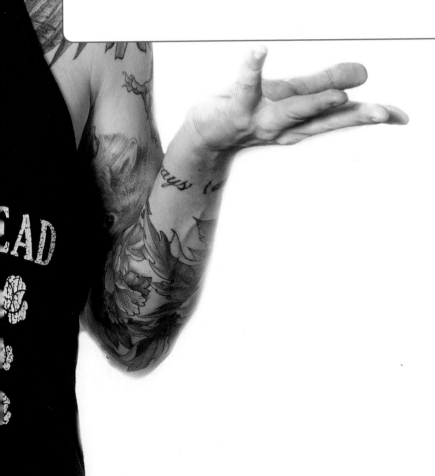

13

Regarding Some Other Lies You Might Have Heard

There's a lot more murkiness in the world of nutrition than just fat-loss programs. We always hear about the latest eating strategy, the newest thing the big pharmaceuticals don't want you to know, and the newest superfoods. (I hate that word, by the way—superfoods aren't usually as super as you think they are. They generally have some really good things about them. But they generally aren't the end-all-be-all they get hyped up to be, but I digress.) And these trends sometimes have a grain of truth—sometimes two or three grains of truth. But usually, they are also a lot of hype and a lot of confusion. This section will clear up some of the topics I get asked about the most.

THE MYTH OF THE ANABOLIC WINDOW

Gym bros have been touting the anabolic window for as long as I can remember. "I gotta down this protein shake *now*," they explain from the weight bench at which they just finished their last set, "or I'll lose all my gains." The anabolic window is some specific time slot directly after training in which carbs and proteins need to be consumed to make whatever work you did in the gym that day really takes effect.

Eating proteins and carbs after an intense training bout serves the purpose of putting glycogen (i.e., muscle fuel) back into your cells. This can be really useful for people who are, for instance, ultra-endurance athletes (and therefore need to refuel during their many hours of exercise), or who train multiple times per day and need to prime their bodies for their next event or workout (107).

Consuming proteins and carbohydrates after training is also thought to help rebuild and repair muscle after training, particularly by spiking insulin levels (insulin can help increase muscle growth). This hasn't really been shown to work as expected in research, though—insulin spiking doesn't seem to affect muscle growth after training that much (107).

For most people, there is no urgent need to refuel muscles in a timely fashion after working out, and neither performance nor physique will really be affected if you wait a few hours after training to eat (107). It's certainly not going to cause a problem to get your protein in right after training, but don't stress out about it too much if that isn't an option. Generally, the time between your pre-workout meal and your post-workout meal should stay within three to four hours if you want to really maximize your results. If you're training while fasting, it's probably a good idea to eat something protein-y and carb-y much sooner after your workout. If you ate a really large protein meal before training, you might be able to go up to six hours between fueling sessions after training. Your body is more concerned about you meeting your daily carb and protein requirements, so unless you have very special athletic or physique goals in which even the tiniest change can make all the difference in the world, make that your priority rather than watching the clock (107).

WHAT ABOUT ORGANIC FOOD?

Most of us associate organic foods with several health benefits—perhaps the food contains more nutrients, or perhaps the use of pesticides has detrimental effects to human health. Many note that organic practices are better for the environment, and many feel that organic foods simply taste better. The organic label comes with a hefty price tag, though. Is it worth the extra cost?

So far, the research doesn't show much of a difference between organic and nonorganic foods in levels of proteins, carbs, or fats. There is some evidence showing that organic produce may be higher in antioxidants and that organic meats and dairy products have healthier fat profiles (such as higher levels of omega-3 fatty acids) (114). There may also be higher levels of some other nutrients (e.g., magnesium, alpha- and beta-carotene, lutein, quercetin, kaempferol, zeaxanthin, some types of fatty acids). Whether or not these differences lead to better health in organic food consumers, though, still needs more investigation.

Organic foods do seem to be lower in not-so-healthy substances such as heavy metals, man-made fertilizers and pesticides, and possibly bacteria that has become resistant to antibiotics (114). While the effects of low-level pesticide residue on human health are currently deemed harmless, this hasn't been determined yet.

Even though synthetic pesticides aren't allowed to be used on certified organic produce, there is still some pesticide residue found on organic products from cross contamination. There are also naturally based pesticides permitted for use in organic farming that are not among the synthetic pesticides tested for in major studies, and the long-term health effects of the allowed levels of these pesticides may be in question, as well (115). Furthermore, some natural pesticides that have been banned in some countries are still eligible to be used on imported produce. Rotneone, for instance, is a naturally derived pesticide that has been found to have harmful health effects and has been banned in the United States. It has not been banned in some countries, however, and imported products from those countries with rotenone are currently still legally considered organic in the United States (116). If you are concerned about pesticide intake, "going organic" may not be the solution.

While organic foods may have higher levels of some nutrients, whether eating organic foods leads to overall better health has not been determined. A bigger factor is the overall quality of the diet and lifestyle. And, let's face it, organic produce is crazy expensive, and it's unrealistic for many people to buy it over the nonorganic stuff. If you forgo fruits and vegetables in order to avoid a perceived danger of conventionally grown produce, your health will probably suffer as a result. The bottom line is that you should eat your fruits and veggies however you can get them. You don't need to go organic to benefit.

WHAT ABOUT GMOS?

The genetic modification of foods (GMOs or GM) is a hot-button topic these days, with a lot of fear-fueled animosity against these types of crops. Many studies have been conducted over the course of the last few decades to determine the safety of genetically modified foods (also called *genetically engineered [GE] foods*). The facts, unfortunately, are kind of muddy.

GMOs have benefits. They can create hardier strains of crops, perhaps reduce reliance on chemical pesticides, increase the nutritional value of foods, and have the potential to help solve nutritional crises in underserved areas of the world. There is plenty of good in the development of new food technology. But the questions about safety remain.

The World Health Organization (WHO) (117) states the following:

GM foods and their safety must be assessed on a case by case basis, making general statements on the safety of all GM foods impossible. GM foods on the international market have passed risk assessments and are not likely to present risks for human health. No effects on human health have been shown as a result of the consumption of such foods by the general population in the countries where they have been approved.

Basically, while the WHO concedes that there is no current evidence that links GMO consumption to human health, this is an ongoing investigation, and there is no way to make a sweeping statement about the general safety of GMO foods.

The National Academies of Sciences, Engineering, and Medicine (118) similarly states the following:

[I]n the absence of long-term, case-controlled studies to examine some hypotheses, the committee examined epidemiological datasets over time from the United States and Canada, where GE food has been consumed since the late 1990s, and similar datasets from the United Kingdom and western Europe, where GE food is not widely consumed. No pattern of differences was found among countries in specific health problems after the introduction of GE foods in the 1990s.

The report essentially says that no health issues have been found in the data collected since GMOs were introduced in the 1990s. The organization also brings up an important issue, though, and that is this:

There have been no long-term, case-controlled human studies performed on the subject of GMOs to date.

This is a major reason why the data here are pretty murky. There has been plenty of research done on animals, and while much of it has demonstrated no effects on the conditions studied, some of it did result in health problems (119). While these results can't necessarily pinpoint genetic modification as the specific reason for the issues, they do leave room for thought. There are also plenty of health conditions that have not been studied, and that leaves room for debate.

Humans aren't mice or rats or pigs, and the results of research on humans may turn out to be quite different. Until these studies have been performed under controlled conditions in humans, it is difficult to come to any conclusions.

Because the data are so inconclusive, it's really hard to say whether or not we need to rail against GMOs. The best I can say is that if you are concerned about the health effects from GMOs, do your best to avoid them when you buy food. However, as in the case of organic foods, this could get expensive and may not be feasible for many people. Be proactive, but not at the expense of eliminating fruits, vegetables, and other healthy foods from your diet, and especially not at the expense of your financial well-being. Like the WHO says, we likely need to take the subject of GMOs on a case-by-case basis, and as more information comes to light, we will be able to make better decisions.

> *There have been no long-term, case-controlled human studies performed on the subject of GMOs to date.*

FRUIT AND LEGUMES ARE NOT THE DEVIL

A lot of the more extreme diet plans like to cut out fruit and legumes. We've touched on this a few times in this book, but I think this is a point worth reiterating.

The main reason given for removing fruit and legumes from the diet is due to their sugar content. I once heard a fairly prominent fitness person claim (and I quote) that "Garbanzo beans are just little sugar bombs." The fact of the matter is that in 100 grams of chickpeas, there are 4.8 grams of sugar (not exactly a bomb's worth). There are also 8.86 grams protein, 7.6 grams fiber, and they are a good source of a host of nutrients such as folate, iron, magnesium, phosphorous, zinc, thiamine, and vitamin B_6 (120). The healthy aspects of garbanzos are nothing to sneeze at, 4.8 grams of sugar be damned.

In one long-term study, people who ate chickpeas were found to also have lower body fat and a lower risk of cardiovascular disease

(120). While this cannot be directly linked to chickpea consumption itself and could be due to chickpea eaters just having a healthier lifestyle in general, we can at least say that the chickpeas didn't seem to contribute much to their weight gain. But why stop at chickpeas? Legumes, in general, have been found to be a pretty darn healthy addition to the diet, providing fiber, complex carbs, and a number of nutrients (which vary depending on the type of bean). One review study noted that replacing high-calorie foods with legumes leads to weight loss (121). Now this isn't due necessarily to some magical ability of beans to burn fat—it simply means that replacing high-calorie foods with beans leads to less energy consumed (and the beans themselves certainly are not causing weight gain).

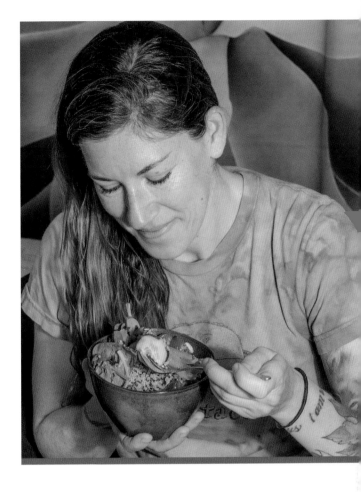

Fruit has a similar story. One of the biggest complaints about fruit is its sugar content. And yes, fruit can serve a rather hefty dose of sugar. That said, fruit also has a ton of healthy nutrients that come along with that, from fiber to different phytochemicals to vitamins, minerals, antioxidants, and more. A higher fruit intake has been linked to lower rates of cancer, heart disease, and, yep, obesity (122). So again, while we can't say that fruit is a direct cause of a reduction in obesity (although there is speculation that some elements of fruit might work against obesity—this is speculation, though, and much more research needs to be done), we can say it likely does not make people fatter on its own. And when it comes down to it, the nutritional reward that fruit delivers outweighs its sugar content.

The bottom line is that you should eat your beans and fruit. Chances are that you'll be healthier for it.

NIGHTSHADES ARE NOT POISON

Nightshades have gotten a bad rap for some reason. The nightshade category includes tomatoes, eggplant, peppers, tomatillos, and potatoes. Tobacco and belladonna are also nightshades, and if those are the night-shades you're concerned about, then let's just go with not consuming tobacco or belladonna. I think that's probably a safe bet.

That said, the other nightshade foods have gotten a pretty bad rap. They've been said to have chemical compounds called *alkaloids*, which can wreak digestive havoc, create inflammation, and aggravate arthritis, among other things. The fact of the matter is, though, that there is no peer-reviewed research demonstrating any of these harmful effects of nightshade vegetables. In fact, there's even a bit of evidence suggesting that compounds in nightshade vegetables may help alleviate arthritis pain to some degree (123).

Furthermore, nightshades are full of some very healthy stuff. The lycopene in tomatoes has been known to reduce risk of prostate cancer and heart disease, among other chronic illnesses, and tomatoes are rich in vitamins A and C (124). Contrary to popular belief, potatoes are not associated with weight gain, diabetes, or heart disease (unless you eat them in fried form, that is) (125). With the skins on, they are good sources of potassium, vitamin C, vitamin B_6, manganese, thiamin, niacin, folate, pantothenic acid, and iron and even provide some protein (126). Eggplants are full of fiber and are a source of manganese, folate, potassium, vitamin K, and vitamin C. They also contain a chemical called anthocyanin, which makes their skin purple and has been shown to help protect against cancers and cardiovascular disease, improve eye health, and help kill bacteria (127). Peppers are great sources of vitamin C, vitamin A, potassium, fiber, and folic acid. In hot peppers, capsaicin, the chemical that packs the heat, has been shown to protect against different types of cancers such as prostate cancer and melanoma, and has anti-inflammatory effects as well (128). Suffice to say, you would be missing out if you decided to take nightshade foods out of your diet.

That said, if you feel better when you don't eat them, by all means, you don't have to eat nightshades. There are plenty of other fruits and vegetables in the world, and there are plenty of benefits to be had from eating those too.

Neither Are Anti-Nutrients

Anti-nutrients has been a buzzword in the world of nutrition, and has been used to demonize plant-based eating and even to claim that vegetables aren't healthy to eat (which is becoming a more and more popular, if niche, viewpoint, even though it is well accepted in science that vegetables are, in fact, extremely healthful and important to eat).

Anti-nutrients is a term used to describe compounds that keep the body from absorbing nutrients. The following anti-nutrients have been demonized:

- Lectins (found in just about every edible plant out there)
- Phytates (found in seeds, beans, and grains)
- Tannins (found in tea, wine, berries, apples, nuts, and beans, to name a few)
- Calcium oxalate (found in many veggies, especially leafy greens, such as spinach)
- Saponins (found mainly in beans, but also in garlic, onion, oats, and more)
- Amylase inhibitors (found mostly in grains and beans)
- Alkaloids (found in nightshades, cocoa, coffee, honey, tea, and black pepper)
- Protease inhibitors (found in most edible plants, and in seeds, beans, and grains in particular)

It is true that anti-nutrients can inhibit certain nutrients and potentially cause other problems. Lectins have been at the root of kidney bean poisoning (that's right—kidney bean poisoning) from undercooked red kidney beans, which have extremely high concentrations of active lectins (129). High doses of lectins can cause stomach distress, fever, and kidney dehydration (129), so this can certainly be problematic.

Phytates can interfere with the absorption of minerals like calcium and magnesium (130). Tannins can interfere with the body's ability to process protein and iron (130). Oxalates can bind with calcium, iron, and magnesium in the body and make those nutrients unavailable, as well as cause stomach discomfort (130). Saponins have gotten a bad rap from seemingly being toxic to fish, rats, and other animals; however, they do not appear to be toxic to humans in normal amounts (129-130). In large doses, saponins might cause some an upset stomach (131). Protease inhibitors may interfere with protein digestion and, in some studies, have been suspected to cause pancreatic cancer (130), and amylase inhibitors can interfere with the digestion of carbs (132). Alkaloids can have cancer-causing qualities and may cause cell mutations (133).

Scary stuff, huh? But there's also a really good side to all of these anti-nutrients. Alkaloids, for instance, have been used in medicine (morphine, codeine, camptothecin, atropine, vinblastine, etc.) as anti-cancer, anti-poison, analgesics, and tranquillizers (134). Everyone's favorite, caffeine, is also an alkaloid. It's been shown to have potential benefits for sport performance, and possibly can improve mood and memory (135). Saponins, lectins, phytates, tannins, and protease inhibitors all seem to have impressive cancer-fighting power (131-132, 136-138). And the fact of the matter is that the foods containing anti-nutrients, for the most part, are extremely nutrient dense and have a host of health benefits. Cutting them out of your diet isn't a great idea for the majority of the population.

There are ways to reduce anti-nutrients in foods, should you wish to do so. Rinsing, sprouting, soaking, fermenting, and heating (or boiling) foods can go a long way in eliminating some of the anti-nutrient content of foods (139-142), and combining some of these methods can be even more effective. Methods such as sprouting and fermenting can also increase the nutrient availability and digestibility of grains and legumes, which is a pretty good side effect (140).

The bottom line is that while some people may experience health problems from anti-nutrients, most healthy humans will be just fine and will reap a lot of benefits from eating the foods that contain anti-nutrients. If you don't react well to certain foods, you can eliminate those foods or try some of the cooking methods that reduce anti-nutrients. But for the most part, carry on.

PINK HIMALAYAN SALT IS NOT BETTER FOR YOU THAN ANY OTHER KIND OF SALT

Pink Himalayan salt is a pink-hued salt mined—guess where—in the Himalayas (specifically in the Khewra Salt Mine in Pakistan). The salt's pinkish color comes from its mineral content, and it is this mineral content that feeds claims that the salt is beneficial to human health.

While it is true that the human body needs a certain amount of sodium to function properly, there is absolutely no scientific evidence that consuming Himalayan salt over regular table salt is beneficial at all. The mineral content of Himalayan salt is higher than that of table salt, so those claims are absolutely true. Proponents of pink salt boast that it has up to 84 different minerals. That is an impressive number, but many of those nutrients are not usable to the human body (and some could be downright harmful) (110).

Himalayan salt certainly also contains valuable minerals, and definitely in higher quantities than table salt. While table salt only has about .9 milligrams of potassium, 1.06 milligrams of magnesium, and 0.4 milligrams of calcium, pink Himalayan salt has 2.8 milligrams, 1.06 milligrams, and 1.6 milligrams, respectively (111). That is all well and good, but these are still incredibly small amounts, and it would take a whole heck of a lot of Himalayan salt to even approach the needed amounts of these minerals. The United States recommended a calcium dosage for men and women between ages 18 and 50 of about 1,000 milligrams (112). A reasonable dose of Himalayan salt isn't going to make much of a dent in that.

The claim that pink Himalayan salt is lower in sodium than table salt is also true—pink Himalayan salt has 368 milligrams of sodium compared to table salt's 381 milligrams (111). The difference isn't huge, so you're really not cutting your sodium intake much by making the switch to the pink stuff.

One benefit table salt has over gourmet salts like pink salt is that it is often enriched with iodine. Many people do not consume enough iodine in their diets, and iodized salt is a good way to get those numbers in check. Unless you're eating seaweed, fish, dairy products, and iodine-enriched foods, iodized salt may be a necessity to avoid iodine deficiency (113).

aLKaLINE DIETS DON'T DO WHAT YOU THINK THEY DO

A common topic I hear in discussions of nutrition is that of the alkaline diet. The theory is that certain foods, particularly those high in protein (and animal protein in particular), causes the body to become more acidic and therefore susceptible to bone loss (osteoporosis), cancer, and other maladies. Proponents of the diet generally test the acidity of the urine to determine how acidic or alkaline the body is in response to the diet.

Here's the thing, though—the body has different pH (a measure of acidity) levels for different areas. The pH scale runs from 0.0 to 14.0, with acidic values running below 7.0, neutral values at 7.0, and alkaline values from 7.1 and up. The stomach is full of stomach acid, so it's pretty acidic, with a pH of anywhere from 1 to 5, depending on what it is digesting at the time. Blood pH is a much narrower window, with a pH of 7.36 to 7.44 (143). Anything beyond this range can prove deadly.

The body is pretty good at maintaining a good acid-base balance. One major way it does this is through the urine. So while food is almost definitely not going to change the pH of your blood in any significant way, it can change the pH of your pee (144). Lots of things can change the pH of your pee, actually, including illness, medication, and even the time of day. But I digress. My point is that when your urine is more acidic or more alkaline, it is not a reflection of the acidity or alkalinity of the rest of your body, and it does not even necessarily reflect your food's effect on your body.

Regarding bone loss, there is currently no convincing evidence to link an acidic diet to osteoporosis (144-145). An alkaline diet is said to cause less calcium excretion in the urine, and that the calcium excreted in the urine comes from bone. However, there is no research that links the calcium excreted in urine to loss of bone breakdown (144-145).

There also doesn't seem to be much of a link between the alkaline diet and cancer (146). While it may be true that cancer cells can grow faster in an acidic environment (146), the fact of the matter is that the blood is not conducive to that acidic state (only the urine becomes acidic in its effort to maintain homeostasis). Cancers can also grow in alkaline environments so an acidic environment is not necessary for cancer growth (151). That said, if we presume that cancer is more prevalent in an acidic environment, it may be possible that the acidity of the urinary tract is more affected by dietary changes, so the alkaline diet might be useful in cancers in that area. It would still need to be proven that acidity is the culprit, though, and that is questionable. In fact, cancer cells seem to create their own acidic environment (152). If cancer creates an acidic environment, then the cause of the acidity could be the cancer, and not the environment.

While there is currently no research on the alkaline diet's effect on urinary tract cancer, there is some evidence that an alkaline diet might be useful in kidney disease (147-150). Kidney disease can lead to a condition called *metabolic acidosis,* in which the kidneys aren't doing their job of regulating the body's acid-base balance through urine. In this case, the body starts to become acidic, which, as we know, can be deadly. Some studies demonstrate that an alkaline diet can help keep acidosis in check and help preserve muscle mass in people affected by the disease (147-150). Taking sodium bicarbonate (baking soda) also seems to do the trick. While a lot more research needs to be done, generally, if the alkaline diet is useful for any disease prevention or treatment at all, it's likely the diseases of the areas involved in producing and excreting urine.

There are plenty of good things about the alkaline diet, but they don't really have much to do with its alkalinity. The alkaline diet is rich in fruits and veggies, which is usually a good plan. It has very little added sugars and processed snack foods, which makes it a healthier choice. If you're a generally healthy person, you're probably not going to get any benefit from increasing the alkalinity of, or decreasing the acid in, your diet. But if you have chronic kidney disease, it may be worth further consideration. Regardless, if the alkaline diet is what it takes to get you to eat more veggies, have at it.

Neither Does Alkaline Water

Alkaline water is water that has either more alkaline than regular water due to a higher concentration of alkaline minerals or that has been artificially alkalized using an ionizer. Alkaline water, much like an alkaline diet, has been credited with miracles such as slowing the aging process, assisting with weight loss, brain protection, cancer protection, body detoxification, digestive health, and strengthening bones, to name a few.

There have been a few studies here and there that have shown potential benefits for alkaline water. One study found that mice who drank alkaline water had longer lifespans than mice who did not, although the water did not seem to change anything else about their organs or body functions (153). However, these results have not been repeated (or even studied) in humans, so it's not possible to say if alkaline water actually increases one's life span or has any anti-aging capabilities.

A study sponsored by Essentia Water, an alkaline water company, demonstrated that alkaline water might lower blood viscosity in healthy adults after exercise (154). If the blood is less viscous, it flows better, can deliver oxygen better, and can reduce strain on the heart. However, there were differences in blood viscosity between participants from the get-go in this study, and that can certainly interfere with study results. Furthermore, the fact that an alkaline water company paid for this study automatically sets up red flags. It does not necessarily mean that the results aren't valid, but it certainly should make us take a harder look at the study.

A 2011 laboratory study on mouse brain cells showed that alkaline water seemed to keep the cells from dying and showed the ability to protect the cells from degeneration (155). Another study demonstrated that rats with Parkinson's disease who were given zamzam water (a naturally alkaline water that comes from a well in Saudi Arabia) seemed to show some signs of brain regeneration compared to a placebo (although it didn't do as good of a job as Parkinson's disease medication) (156). Again, these results have not been replicated or attempted in humans, so no conclusions can really be made (and then there's that whole thing about not placing all your bets on evidence coming from one small study).

One study out of China showed that blood pressure and blood lipids improved after drinking alkalized water for three to six months (157), and another study found that alkalized water improved blood sugar and blood lipids in rats (158). Interesting information, but once again, a lot more research needs to be done before any recommendations can really be made.

Alkaline water at a pH of 8.8 was useful in the treatment of acid reflux in one study (159). Again, more research is needed on this subject.

The bottom line is that while alkaline water might have some merit, there's really not much evidence in humans demonstrating most of the health claims surrounding it. We also don't know if there could potentially be harmful effects of drinking a lot of alkaline water over the long term. If you feel good drinking alkaline water keep it up. But don't chalk up too many miracles to the stuff.

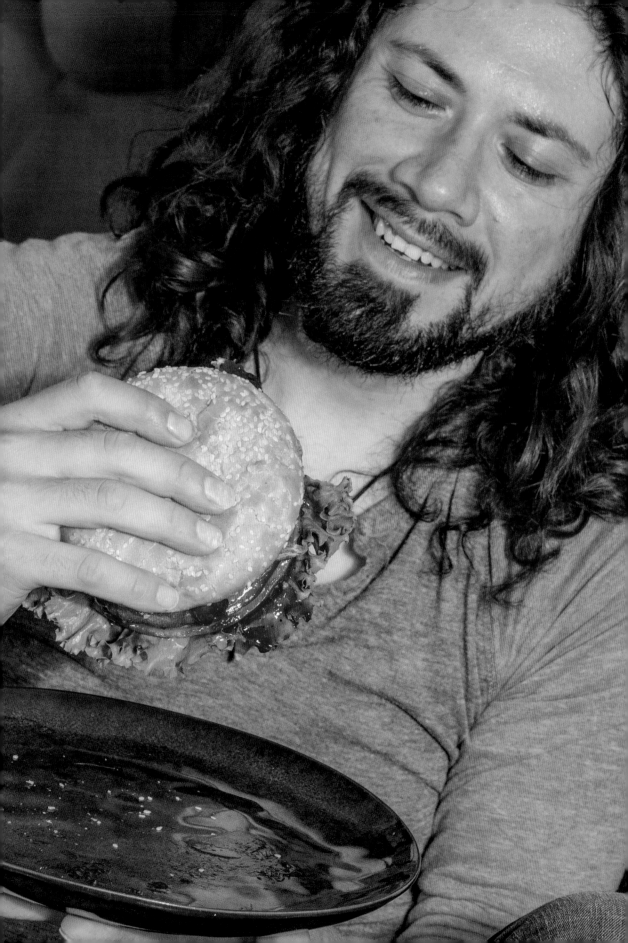

14

So What's the Best Diet?

When it comes down to it, all diets work, more or less. If a diet leads to eating fewer calories than you're burning off, it will probably end up leading to weight loss. The three questions you need to ask yourself, then, are as follows:

1. Do I enjoy this diet?
2. Does this diet keep me healthy?
3. Can I keep doing this diet for maintenance, even after I lose the weight I want to lose?

These are important questions. Most people are unsuccessful at long-term weight loss because the diets they choose make them miserable or are unsustainable long-term. The "best diet" is not a one-size-fits-all equation. The best diet is the one you can stick with for life.

SAMPLE DIETS

To help you figure out what way of eating may work best for you, here are some sample eating plans you may want to try. These are provided by Dr. Susan Kleiner, a registered dietitian.

The key words of successful nutrition are *plan, shop,* and *cook*. It's great to figure out which diet you think will work for you based on the description of the diet, but actually following the diet is a completely different story. You may read about grams, calories, and timing, but you don't eat those; you eat food. So how do you plan a menu that meets those guidelines? Or you may think that the Mediterranean- or vegan-style diet sounds best for you, but how do you get all those foods into your meals and snacks every day? That's where menu planning, shopping, and cooking really count.

Use these sample menu plans to see what a day in the life of the diet really looks like. *Plan* a couple of your own daily menus. What will you need to do to have the food available to prepare those menus? Are there foods that you will need to substitute? Will you need new recipes? Create a shopping list and decide where and how often you will *shop*. We know that the first steps toward successful change depend on having more, rather than less, control over the foods that you eat. This means that at least at the beginning of your diet journey, how often you *cook* for yourself rather than eating out or getting takeout will likely set you up for a more successful outcome.

Mediterranean Diet

Let's start here as kind of a "day in the diet template." I like using the Mediterranean diet as the starting point because it is not based on restriction and has good evidence that it promotes health, as well as an ability to support weight loss when you eat well but don't overdo it.

Each meal plan is based on a daily 2,000-kilocalorie diet.

Hallmarks of the Diet

- It's high in veggies, fruit, whole grains, legumes, herbs and spices, fish, and olive oil.
- Poultry, eggs, and dairy are included more sparingly, and red meat is eaten only occasionally.
- Refined, sugary, and commercially processed meats and snacks are generally avoided in this diet.

Food group serving	Menu
MEAL	
2 breads/starches	1 cup (30 g) whole grain cereal (sugar free)
1 fruit	1/2 cup (90 g) fresh fruit
1 milk	1 cup (240 mL) milk
1 medium-fat protein	1 egg
1 fat	1 tablespoon (9 g) pumpkin (or other) seeds in cereal
MEAL OR SNACK	
1 fruit	1/2 (90 g) cup pineapple
1 milk + 2 proteins	1 cup (230 g) plain Greek yogurt
1 fat	1 tablespoon (9 g) almonds
MEAL	
2 breads/starches + 2 proteins	1 cup (200 g) cooked legumes/beans
2 vegetables	Mixed green salad with herbs
3 very lean proteins	3 ounces (90 g) chicken
1 fat	1 teaspoon (5 g) of olive oil plus vinegar; or 1 tablespoon (15 g) oil and vinegar dressing
MEAL OR SNACK	
1 fruit	Apple
2 vegetables	1 cup (240 mL) vegetable juice
2 very lean proteins + 2 fats	2 ounces (60 g) cheese
MEAL	
2 breads/starches servings	1 cup (200 g) cooked farro with veggies and herbs
1 fruit	Grapes
2 vegetables	Cooked broccoli sprinkled with balsamic vinegar
5 lean proteins	5 ounces (150 g) grilled or broiled wild salmon
2 fats	8 kalamata olives + extra virgin olive oil for salmon

Vegan Diet

Let's take the healthy Mediterranean-style meal plan and make it vegan.

Note: If beans or certain vegetables give you intestinal distress (a little gassy?), try using the product Beano, which is a natural enzyme. It will help you digest beans and vegetables more fully and decrease the side effects that many people experience from beans.

Hallmarks of the Diet

- 100 percent plant-based
- Zero animal-sourced foods

Food group serving	Menu
MEAL	
2 breads/starches	2 slices (2 oz) 100 percent whole grain bread
1 fruit	1/2 sliced banana
1 soy milk	1 cup (240 mL) soy milk
2 high-fat protein	2 tablespoons (32 g) natural peanut butter
MEAL OR SNACK	
1 fruit	1/2 cup (90 g) frozen blueberries
1 almond milk	1 cup (240 mL) almond milk
4 very lean protein	30 grams plant-based protein powder
MEAL	
2 breads/starches + 2 proteins	1 cup (200 g) cooked legumes (e.g., pinto beans)
2 vegetables	Mixed green salad with herbs; add beans to salad
2 proteins	6 ounces (180 g) grilled tofu
1 fat	1 teaspoon (5 g) of olive oil plus vinegar; or 1 tablespoon (15 g) oil and vinegar dressing
MEAL OR SNACK	
2 vegetables	1 cup (30-100 g) raw vegetable sticks
2 very lean proteins + 2 fats	1/2 cup (115 g) hummus
MEAL	
2 breads/starches servings + 2 vegetables + 3 lean proteins	Lentil stew (www.eatingwell.com/recipe/277566/instant-pot-lentil-soup)
2 fats	1/4 avocado
SNACK	
1 breads/starches + 2 lean proteins	1 cup (180 g) edamame in shells

Low-Carbohydrate Diet

Carbohydrates are the primary fuel for our muscles and brain. While it takes a surprising number of calories to fuel brain work, physical activity requires the mother lode of energy needs in a healthy person. During your more sedentary days, you might choose to lower your carbohydrate intake to meet your lower activity needs. This menu plan is low in carbohydrate but still roomy enough to be chock full of vegetables and a little fruit, and not so low that it's painful to follow. A low-carbohydrate diet can be dehydrating, so focus on your fluids!

Hallmark of the Diet

- <100 grams a day of carbohydrate

Food group serving	Menu
	MEAL
	Omelet:
3 medium-fat proteins	2 eggs + 1 ounce (30 g) shredded cheddar cheese
1 very lean protein	2 egg whites
2 fats	1/4 avocado, sliced
Free (no calories)	1 tablespoon (15 g) no-added-sugar salsa
	2 cups water
	MEAL OR SNACK
1 milk + 2 lean proteins	1 cup (230 g) plain low-fat Greek yogurt
1 fruit	1/2 cup (90 g) fresh berries, halved
2 fats	1 ounce (about 2 tablespoons) slivered or sliced almonds
	MEAL
	Large tuna salad:
4 lean proteins	4 ounces (120 g) fresh grilled or canned tuna +
1 medium-fat proteins	1 ounce (30 g) feta cheese, cubed +
3 vegetables	2 cups (56 g) leafy greens + 1/2 cup (81 g) steamed green string beans + 3 red onion rings + 3 cherry tomatoes +
3 fats	5 green olives + 8 kalamata olives + oil and vinegar dressing
	2 cups water

(continued)

Low-Carbohydrate Diet *(continued)*

Food group serving	Menu
MEAL OR SNACK	
1 milk	1 cup (240 mL) nonfat milk
3 very lean proteins	1 scoop (20 grams) whey protein isolate
1 fruit	1/2 cup (90 g) frozen berries
MEAL	
	"Spaghetti" with meatballs:
5 lean proteins	5 ounces (150 g) meatballs
7 vegetables	Sauté 2 cups (328 g) spaghetti squash, shredded + 1/4 cup (41 g) mushrooms + 1/2 cup (81 g) zucchini + garlic + olive oil + 1/2 cup (120 mL) organic, canned, chopped tomatoes in liquid or sauce
	Large salad: 2 cups (60-200 g) mixed greens + 6 sliced radishes + 1 tablespoon fresh chopped parsley + 1 small tomato, sliced
2 fats	grated Parmesan cheese (optional) EVOO and vinegar dressing
	2 cups water

Low Fat Diet

There are a couple of reasons why you might be interested in this diet style. Some research has shown that a 10 percent fat diet may help to reverse certain types of coronary artery disease. Other research has shown that there are clearly some people that sustain a low-fat diet better than a low carbohydrate diet. So if you are trying to figure out where to remove a few extra calories, you might already know whether you feel better with less fat or less carbohydrate. As a starting point, go with that gut instinct.

Hallmark of the Diet

- 10 percent fat per day

Food group serving	Menu
MEAL OR SNACK	
1 milk	1 cup (230 g) plain yogurt
1 fruit	3/4 cup (109 g) blueberries
WORKOUT	
	water
MEAL	
1 bread/starch	1 slice (1 oz) whole-grain bread
1 milk	1 cup (240 mL) fat-free milk
1 fruit	1/2 cup (120 mL) orange juice
1 medium-fat protein	1 whole egg, scrambled in nonstick skillet
5 very lean proteins	4 egg whites, cooked with whole egg, 21 grams whey protein isolate, blended with milk, orange juice, and 3 or 4 ice cubes
MEAL OR SNACK	
1 vegetable	1 cup (124 g) celery sticks
2 lean proteins + 1 breads/starches	1 cup (180 g) edamame (in shells) or 2 servings (about 2/3 bag) of soy crisps
MEAL	
4 breads/starches	6-inch Subway turkey breast sandwich
2 vegetables	Fill with vegetable choices
4 very lean proteins	4 ounces (120 g) turkey (request extra turkey to make 4 oz)
Free (no calories)	Dijon mustard (no mayo or oil)
MEAL OR SNACK	
1 fruit	4 dried apricots
1 milk	1 tall nonfat latté
MEAL	
2 breads/starches	1 baked sweet potato
3 vegetable	1/2 cup (90 g) steamed asparagus 4 cups (112 g) mixed green salad with balsamic vinegar for dressing
8 lean proteins	8 ounces (240 g) wild salmon, grilled

Intermittent Fasting

This is basically the practice of going without food, or at least undereating, for a specified period of time on a regular basis. If you are skipping food altogether for 24 hours, then you don't need a diet plan guide. However, the 16/8 method limits eating to about eight hours per day, with fasting taking place the rest of the day. There is some leeway with the fasting hours and eating hours, with some people fasting using 14/10, 15/9, 18/6, or some other variation on this theme. This essentially works out to skipping a meal (breakfast or dinner, usually). The eight-ish hours you spend asleep after dinner can help the fasting go a little easier. This guideline takes the Mediterranean diet and works it into a 14/10 plan.

You might find that reducing the number of meals and snacks works better within the hours that you have allotted for eating. Just combine the foods into fewer meals and the plan will work just as well for you. Finish dinner the night before by 5:30 p.m. Eat breakfast at 7:30 a.m.

Hallmark of the Diet

- Going without food, or at least undereating, for a specified period of time on a regular basis

Food group serving	Menu
MEAL OR SNACK AT 7:30 A.M.	
2 breads/starches	1 cup (30 g) whole-grain cereal
1 fruit	1/2 cup (90 g) fresh fruit
1 milk	1 cup (240 mL) milk
1 medium-fat protein	1 egg
1 fat	1 tablespoon (9 g) pumpkin (or other) seeds in cereal
SNACK AT 10:00 A.M.	
1 fruit	1/2 cup (90 g) pineapple
1 milk + 2 proteins	1 cup (230 g) plain Greek yogurt
1 fat	1 tablespoon (9 g) almonds
MEAL AT 12:30 P.M.	
2 breads/starches + 2 proteins	1 cup (200 g) cooked legumes/beans
2 vegetables	Mixed green salad with herbs
3 very lean proteins	3 ounces (90 g) chicken
1 fat	1 teaspoon (5 g) of olive oil plus vinegar; or 1 tablespoon (15 g) oil and vinegar dressing
SNACK AT 3:00 P.M.	
1 fruit	Apple
2 vegetables	1 cup (240 mL) vegetable juice
2 very lean proteins + 2 fats	2 ounces (60 g) cheese
MEAL AT 5:00 P.M.	
2 bread servings	1 cup (200 g) cooked farro with veggies and herbs
1 fruit	Grapes
2 vegetable	Cooked broccoli sprinkled with balsamic vinegar
5 lean proteins	5 ounces (150 g) grilled or broiled wild salmon
2 fats	8 kalamata olives + extra virgin olive oil for salmon

KNOWING YOUR PORTIONS

A portion is the amount of food used to determine the numbers of servings for each food group; it is the physical measurement of one serving. The amount of food that makes up a portion is not usually what you would think of as a serving, however. For example, one portion of cooked pasta is just a half cup (70 g). If you have pasta for dinner, you would likely eat at least 1 cup (140 g), but since one serving is a half cup, one cup of pasta equals two servings from the bread and starch group. Learning the portion sizes for servings is the foundation of success when counting macros (see tables 14.1 through 14.6).

Table 14.1   Milk and Yogurt Group

Each portion contains 90 to 110 calories, 8 grams protein, and 12 grams carbohydrate.

Food	Size of one portion
Nonfat or low-fat milk	1 cup (240 mL)
Evaporated nonfat milk	1 cup (240 mL)
Nonfat dry milk powder	1/3 cup (22 g)
Plain nonfat yogurt	1 cup (230 g)
Plain nonfat Greek yogurt	6 ounces (173 g)
Nonfat or low-fat soy or rice milk, fortified with calcium and vitamins A and D	1 cup (240 mL)

Reprinted by permission from S.M. Kleiner with M. Greenwood-Robinson, *The New Power Eating* (Champaign, IL: Human Kinetics, 2019), 271.

Table 14.2   Vegetable Group

Each portion contains approximately 25 calories, 2 grams protein, and 5 grams carbohydrate.

Food	Size of one portion
Most cooked vegetables	1/2 cup (81 g)
Most raw vegetables	1 cup (30-100 g)
Raw lettuce	2 cups (56 g)
Sprouts	1 cup (30 g)
Vegetable juice	6 ounces (180 mL)
Vegetable soup	1 cup (240 mL)
Tomato sauce	1/2 cup (120 mL)
Salsa (made without oil)	3 tablespoons (45 g)

Reprinted by permission from S.M. Kleiner with M. Greenwood-Robinson, *The New Power Eating* (Champaign, IL: Human Kinetics, 2019), 272.

Table 14.3   Fruit Group

Each portion contains about 60 calories and 15 grams carbohydrate.

Food	Size of one portion
Most fruits, whole	1 medium
Most fruits, chopped or canned in own juice	1/2 cup (120 g)
Melon, diced	1 cup (156 g)
Berries, cherries, or grapes (whole)	3/4 cup (80 g)
Fruit juice	1/2 cup (120 mL)
Banana	1 small
Grapefruit or mango	1/2 cup
Plums	2 medium
Apricots	4 medium
Strawberries, whole	1 1/4 cup (180 g)
Kiwi	1 medium
Prunes, dried	3 medium
Figs	2 medium
Raisins	2 tablespoons (28 g)
Juice: cranberry, grape, or fruit blends (100% juice)	1/3 cup (80 mL)
Cranberry juice cocktail (reduced calorie)	1 cup (240 mL)

Reprinted by permission from S.M. Kleiner with M. Greenwood-Robinson, *The New Power Eating* (Champaign, IL: Human Kinetics, 2019), 272.

Table 14.4   Bread and Starch Group

Each portion contains 60 to 100 calories, 2-3 grams protein, 15 grams carbohydrate, ≤1 gram fat.

Food	Size of one portion
Bread	1 slice (1 oz)
Pita	1 small (1 oz)
Bagel, English muffin, or bun	1/2 small (1 oz)
Roll	1 small
Cooked rice or cooked pasta	1/2 cup (97 g)
Tortilla	6 inch round (15 cm)
Crackers, large	2 large or 3 or 4 small
Croutons	1/3 cup (13 g)
Pretzels or baked chips	1 ounce (30 g)
Rice cakes	2
Cooked cereal	1/2 cup (119 g)
Cold cereal, unsweetened	1/2-1 cup (15-30 g)
Granola	1/2 cup (30 g)
Corn, green peas, or mashed potatoes	1/2 cup (105 g)
Corn on the cob	1 medium
White or sweet potato baked with skin	1 small
Plantain, sliced and cooked	1/3 cup (39 g)

Reprinted by permission from S.M. Kleiner with M. Greenwood-Robinson, *The New Power Eating* (Champaign, IL: Human Kinetics, 2019), 273.

Table 14.5 Protein Group

Each protein portion contains about 35 to 75 calories and 7 grams of protein. Very lean servings contain 35 calories and 0 to 1 gram of fat; lean, 55 calories and 3 grams of fat; medium-fat, 75 calories and 5 grams of fat; and high-fat, 100 calories and 8 grams of fat.

Food	Size of one portion
VERY LEAN	
White meat skinless poultry	1 ounce (30 g)
White fish	1 ounce (30 g)
Fresh or canned tuna in water	1 ounce (30 g)
All shellfish	1 ounce (30 g)
Beans, peas, or lentils*	1/2 cup (100 g)
Cheeses and processed sandwich meat with 1 g of fat	1 ounce (30 g)
Egg whites	2
LEAN	
Select or choice grades of lean beef, pork, lamb, or veal trimmed to 0 fat	1 ounce (30 g)
Dark-meat skinless poultry or white-meat chicken with skin	1 ounce (30 g)
Oysters, salmon, catfish, sardines, or tuna canned in oil	1 ounce (30 g)
Cheese and deli sandwich meat with 3 g of fat	1 ounce (30 g)
Parmesan cheese	1 ounce (30 g)
MEDIUM-FAT	
Dark-meat poultry with skin or most styles of beef, pork, lamb, or veal, trimmed of fat	1 ounce (30 g)
Ground turkey or chicken	1 ounce (30 g)
Cheese with 5 g of fat	1 ounce (30 g)
Cottage cheese, 4.5% fat	1/4 cup (56 g)
Whole egg	1 large
Tempeh	4 ounces or 1/2 cup (120 g)
Tofu	4 ounces or 1/2 cup (120 g)
HIGH-FAT VEGETARIAN	
All regular cheese: American, Swiss, cheddar	1 ounce (30 g)
Natural peanut butter	1 tablespoon (16 g)

*One portion counts as one very lean protein and one starch.

Reprinted by permission from S.M. Kleiner with M. Greenwood-Robinson, *The New Power Eating* (Champaign, IL: Human Kinetics, 2019), 273-274.

Table 14.6 Fats and Oils Group

Each portion contains about 45 calories and 5 grams of fat.

Food	Size of one portion
Butter or margarine	1 teaspoon (5 g)
Cream cheese, cream, or sour cream	1 tablespoon (15 g)
Cream cheese, whipped cream, or sour cream (low fat)	2 tablespoons (30 g)
Salad dressing (full fat)	1 tablespoon (15 g)
Salad dressing (low fat or nonfat)	1 tablespoon (15 g)
Avocado	1/8 medium (2 tablespoons, 30 g)
Olives, black	8 large
Nuts	6-10
Seeds	1 tablespoon (9 g)
Peanut butter or other nut butters	1/2 tablespoon (8 g)

Reprinted by permission from S.M. Kleiner with M. Greenwood-Robinson, *The New Power Eating* (Champaign, IL: Human Kinetics, 2019), 274.

Here's how it works in practice. Let's say you want a diet that is 2,000 calories and 40:30:30 from carbohydrate:protein:fat. This refers to the percentage of macronutrients per total daily calories. But you ultimately need to determine your macros in gram weight so you can figure out your food plan. You start with calories and work back to macronutrient grams.

1 gram carbohydrate = 4 calories

1 gram protein = 4 calories

1 gram fat = 9 calories

1. Determine your total daily calories.
2. Determine the total percentage of calories from each macronutrient.
3. Divide the daily macronutrient calories by number of calories per gram.
4. Now you have the number of grams per macronutrient you want to eat each day.

Once you do the math for a 2,000-calorie diet you can see that your meal plan goals are to have 200 grams of carbohydrate, 150 grams of protein, and 67 grams of fat. Create a spreadsheet with a distribution of food groups that result in these goals. While it's easy to achieve your goals using only two or three food groups, that's not the healthiest strategy. Distribute your macros and calories from among all of the food groups to gain the greatest nutritional advantage. For example, while you may eliminate animal foods as a vegan, you should still consume plant foods from the protein-rich group. You should include gluten-free whole grains, even if you are designing a gluten-free diet. Dairy-free diets with the purpose of managing lactose-intolerance are the most well rounded when lactose-free dairy is consumed, or you can use a lactase-replacement enzyme to support dairy in your diet.

How to Count Macros

The simplest way to learn how to count macros in your head is to learn the macronutrient distributions based on food groups. Originally created for use by dietitians to help diabetic patients manage carb consumption and total food consumption, the classic food group (macronutrient) distribution system is used worldwide as an easy, "back of the napkin" calculation to keep track of your macros.

The macronutrient content of the foods within the food group is relative to the standardized portion sizes. The portion sizes are used only as a way of creating a useful system. You are not required to serve your own portions based on these amounts. For instance, a standard single serving of pasta is a half cup. You may prefer to eat one cup. You can determine your macronutrient intake by doubling the macronutrients in the chart listed under the bread/starch food group for two servings of pasta.

Once you learn the grams of protein, fat, and carbohydrate in each food group portion, you can plan meals by calculating your macros from each food group based on your desired distribution. Be aware that when you focus only on counting macros you may minimize the variety in your diet.

> *Variety is absolutely essential to the framework of a healthy diet.*

Select foods from all the food groups to ensure a healthy variety of micronutrients, phytochemicals, fibers, and all the other factors in whole foods, in addition to their macronutrients. Table 14.7 lists nutrients and calories per single serving.

Table 14.7　Nutrients Per Food Group Single Portion Serving

Food groups	Carbohydrate (g)	Protein (g)	Fat (g)	Calories
Bread/starch	15	3	1 or less	72-81
Fruit	15	—	—	60
Nonfat milk	12	8	0-1	80-89
Low-fat milk	12	8	3	107
Vegetables	5	2	—	25
Very lean protein	—	7	0-1	35
Lean protein	—	7	3	55
Medium-fat protein	—	7	5	75
Fat	—	—	5	45

Reprinted by permission from S.M. Kleiner with M. Greenwood-Robinson, *The New Power Eating* (Champaign, IL: Human Kinetics, 2019), 270. Adapted from American Diabetes Association and American Dietetic Association, Exchange Lists for Meal Planning (Alexandria, VA: American Diabetes Association, 1995).

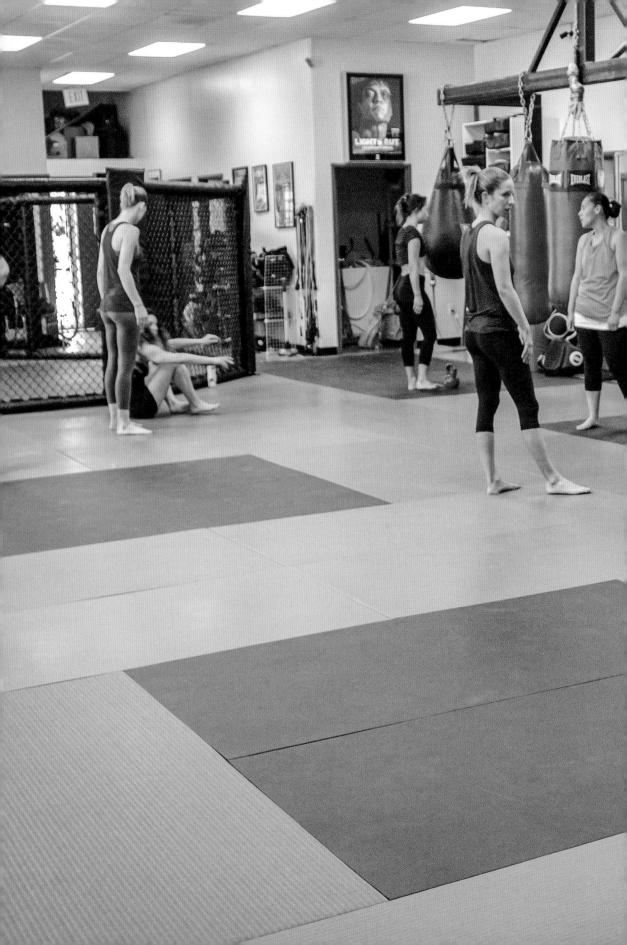

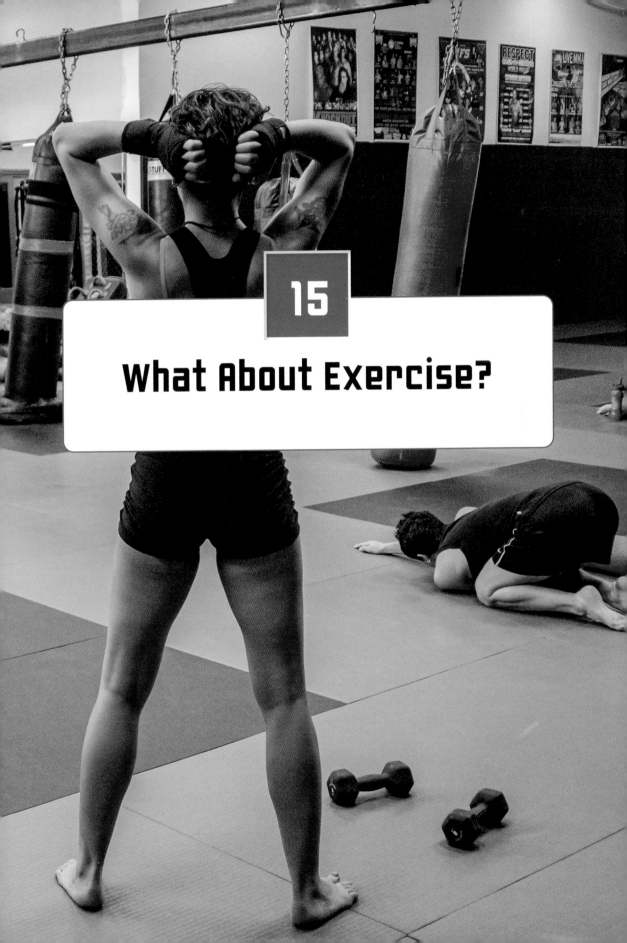

15

What About Exercise?

So you've found a diet plan you like: It's financially doable; you like the food; it doesn't hinder social events, make you feel deprived, or make you hate life; and it seems like something you could feasibly maintain ongoing. That. Is. Awesome. But, of course, it is not the only piece of the puzzle.

YOU GOTTA MOVE

If you really want to sustainably lose weight, dieting is awesome. But you should also add movement. While dieting alone can be effective at helping people lose weight, adding exercise is more effective at lowering visceral fat, which is the fat lying over the organs in your abdomen (i.e., your liver, intestines, stomach, and perhaps inside your arteries as well), and is a better predictor of disease risk and early death (160, 166). So clearly, exercise is an extremely important component of fat loss and overall health. But what's the right exercise plan?

What Are You Willing to Do?

Frankly, I don't care what kind of physical activity you choose, just so long as it gets you moving. Do you love dancing? Take a dance class, go to a Zumba class, or boogie down to something groovy in your living room for 30 minutes. Do you like bouncing around? Take a trampoline or kangaroo jumps class. Are you into circus stuff? Learn how to do rings, silks, or other aerial arts. Are you old-school? Pull out those Jane Fonda or Richard Simmons tapes and have at it. Feel like hitting something? Take a boxing, kickboxing, or martial arts class; or take a sledgehammer to a big tire for a while. Love the water? Go swimming, canoeing, kayaking, surfing, snorkeling, or scuba diving. Like the outdoors? Take a walk, take a hike, take a run, go bouldering, play with your kids, or play with your dog. Like the indoors more? Play Wii or *Dance Dance Revolution*, hop on a stationary bike or elliptical trainer, or do lunges and pushups in your bedroom. Anything that gets you moving will be way better than couch potato–ing and will at least burn some calories. Plus, if you enjoy your physical activity, you're more likely to stick with it.

That said, there are certainly ways to train that are more effective for fat loss than others.

High Intensity Versus Moderate Intensity?

There's a lot of hype about high-intensity interval training (HIIT) these days, and it certainly does pack a punch. HIIT is pretty much what it sounds like—extremely high-intensity bursts of exercise (about 90 percent of your max capacity) followed by shorter rest periods. It can be done with strength training exercises, as well as cardiovascular exercises—so, for instance, you might sprint for 40 seconds, then rest for 20 seconds, then do pushups for 40 seconds, then rest for 20 seconds, and so on. Moderate-intensity continuous training, on the other hand, is done at a more—guess what—moderate pace, and it's done without the rest periods. So you might bike for 30 minutes (with a short warm-up and cool-down) at about 60 percent of your max, or you might do more moderate-intensity strength exercises all in a row for 30 minutes.

In the research that has been done to date on high-intensity training versus moderate-intensity continuous training, both do a pretty job of reducing fat and shrinking waistlines, and one does not actually seem to be better than the other for fat loss *percentage* (161-162). That said, HIIT does seem to get better results for *absolute* fat loss (i.e., total grams of fat lost) (162), so keep that in mind.

If you're just starting out with exercise, you might be better off going the moderate intensity route. If you're not ready for HIIT, you might not be able to perform at a high-enough intensity to get the benefits from it, and it may involve movements at a more advanced skill level that you might not be able to execute properly. This means you'll be frustrated, possibly injured, and might feel like a failure. None of this is enjoyable, and chances are you'll quit. The main kind of exercise that has absolutely no benefit is the one you don't do, so don't go the route that makes you quit. Moderate-intensity training is a great choice for you.

> *Do what works for you now, and when you need more, add more.*

Then again, HIIT doesn't take quite as much time to finish, and a lot of people might find that aspect appealing. There is also a pretty big contingent of people that need to be really drenched in sweat and out of breath after a workout in order to feel as if they've accomplished anything, and for those people, HIIT can bring some peace of mind. Some people simply love higher-intensity exercise, so if that describes you, HIIT might be the way to go. HIIT also seems to have greater cardiovascular health benefits than moderate training for both healthy people and people with heart disease, as well as better benefits for lowering blood pressure and fasting blood sugar levels in obese people (161-162). With those benefits in mind, it might be worth it to try to work your way up to HIIT. If it's not something you can stick with over time, though, it's better to do what you're willing to do than nothing at all.

It's worth noting that there isn't a set way to perform HIIT or moderate-intensity training, so it's hard to say how to do either one the absolute best way. The best advice I can give you for now is to do what you are able to without pain, and don't push yourself so hard that you get turned off to training altogether. Do what works for you now, and when you need more, add more.

Strength Training Versus Cardio

There has always been a sort of battle between the camps of endurance training and weight training about who has the best edge over fat loss. Who's right? The answer is, of course, "it depends."

I want to say so, so badly that strength training wins out over cardio for fat loss. I'm a strength athlete, personally, and I know I've seen the best improvements in my own physique since I started powerlifting and strongman training. I love me some weights. But alas, the research simply does not echo my sentiments. Cardiovascular activity seems to be the winner when it comes to losing body fat (163-165). Furthermore, cardiovascular exercise appears to outperform weight training when it comes to getting rid of visceral fat as well (165). As I mentioned earlier, visceral fat is pretty dangerous stuff—it can be a major predictor of type 2 diabetes, different kinds of cancers, cardiovascular disease, and more (166); cardiovascular activity seems to be key to getting rid of some of the stuff (165). What's more, adding weight training to cardio doesn't really seem to improve fat-loss results of any kind over cardio alone (163-165).

That said, don't write off weight training just yet. Let's talk about lean mass. Lean mass is basically everything in your body that isn't fat,

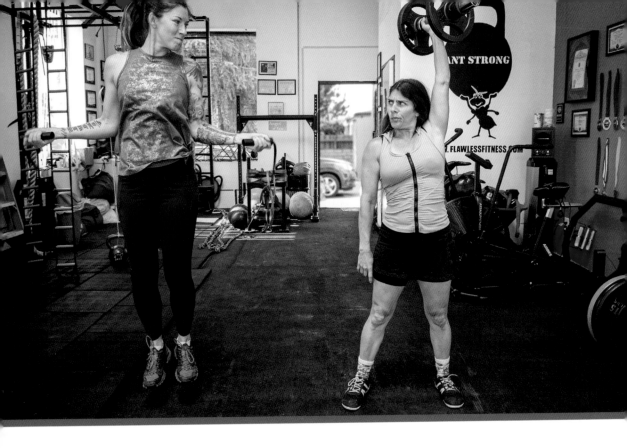

including organs, water, and so on. For our purposes, we will be discussing the muscle portion of your lean body mass, as I'm not sure there are too many exercises that will increase the weight of your organs. Resistance training increases lean body mass far better than aerobic training does (163-167). When people are in a caloric deficit, some muscle is often lost alongside fat. Resistance training helps to preserve muscle mass, while aerobic exercise isn't particularly useful in that respect. Resistance training also helps increase bone density and muscular strength far more than aerobic exercise does (167). Lean mass, physical strength, and bone strength are critical for health, independence, and longevity, so don't underestimate the importance of this component.

Because muscle is denser than fat, you might find that you weigh more than you think you should once you put on some muscle. While that can be frustrating to see, pay attention to what you see in the mirror more than the scale's numbers, as you will probably like what you see when you add lean mass.

To sum it all up, cardiovascular activity seems to be better for reducing fat, while strength training is superior for increasing lean mass. Do both and reap all the benefits.

Fasted Training: Yah or Nah?

Contrary to popular belief, you don't have to train on an empty stomach to increase fat loss from training—the science simply doesn't support a fat loss advantage of fasted training over fed training (209). Most people also don't perform as well when they don't have a good fuel source to work off of, so chances are, you won't be able to work out as intensely. You're likely better off having eaten something at least an hour or two before working out.

If you get nauseous when you eat before training, you might want to look into eating something kinder to your stomach. Play around with different kinds of protein and carb sources and ratios and see which work best for you. If you still get nauseous, you might need a bigger window between eating and training.

If you love training on no food, more power to you—keep doing what works for you. Just know that it isn't going to make you a fat-burning machine.

NO TIME TO WORK OUT?

If you don't have, say, 45 minutes to set aside to train (or don't have the patience to do it all at once), don't fret too much. You can get similar results by breaking up the same amount of time and intensity of exercise into smaller bouts throughout the day (185). So you can, for instance, bang out four 10-minute sweat sessions and one 5-minute session here and there between the time you wake up and the time you go to bed, or whatever fits your schedule.

One little trick I like to give my clients is a 200-rep challenge to do daily. By the end of the day, they need to finish 200 reps of some kind of physical activity involving big muscle groups (i.e., some kind of squat or lunge, some kind of pushing movement, some kind of pulling movement, some kind of hip hinge like a deadlift or kettlebell swing). So, for instance, in the morning a client can do 10 pushups, 10 situps, and 10 squats. Right before leaving the house, the client can do 10 lunges on each leg (that's 20!) and 10 more pushups. During lunch break, a client might do 10 side lunges per leg, 20 more squats, and 10 triceps dips. That's 110 reps by lunchtime! What this does is give a client a goal and make them aware of making physical activity a manageable part of their day. You can also try a 45-minute challenge (i.e., a complete 45 minutes of cardio by end of day), or something similar. Whatever method you choose, you can absolutely make physical activity work within your schedule; you just need to find a few minutes sprinkled throughout the day to make it happen.

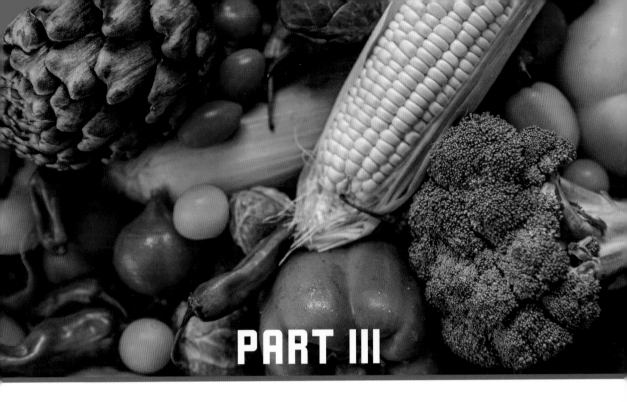

PART III

But what about all the other stuff? It all sounds so easy, doesn't it? Eat less than you burn off and move your body. That's pretty much the whole equation, isn't it? Well, no, not even close. Because, honestly, if it was that easy, no one would ever sell a diet book again, and obesity epidemics would be a thing of the past. The fact of the matter is that fat loss is pretty complicated. There are biological, genetic, and psychological components that make things a lot murkier, and everyone has their own Mt. Everest to climb when it comes to fat loss.

I wanted to cover as much ground as possible in this section, so I turned to the experts—my social media followers—and asked them what their obstacles to fat loss have been. I got lots and lots of answers. Eight hours in, the thread was up to 90 comments and counting. Many of the respondents had similar answers, and some had answers unique to them. On the following pages, I will try to address all the obstacles presented to me in that thread, plus those I see every day with my own clients. Hopefully by the end of it, you'll have a better idea of how you might be able to tackle some of these roadblocks or at least get a better understanding of why they are getting in your way.

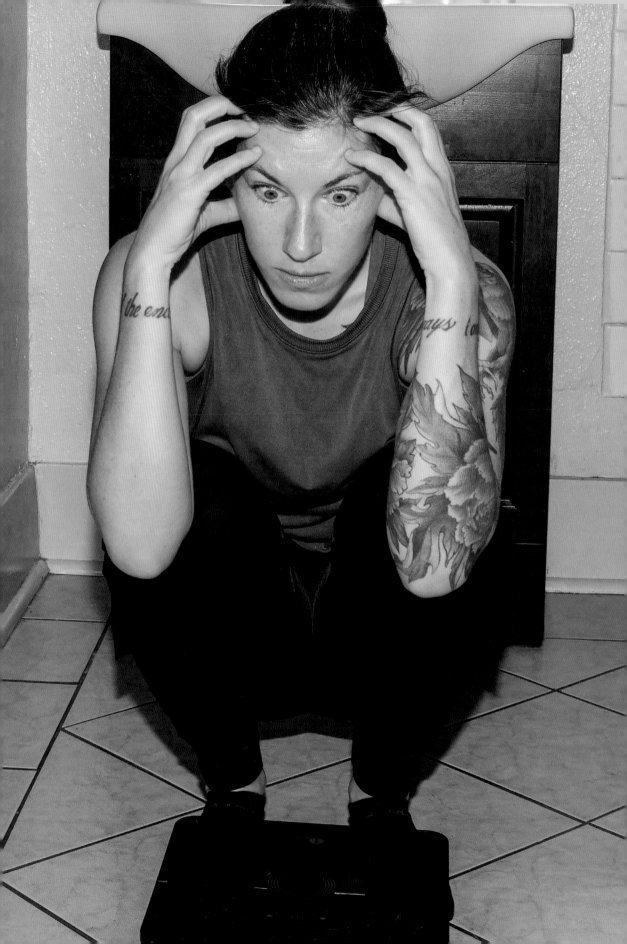

16

Biology and Weight Loss

Sometimes our bodies won't do what we want them to do, even when it seems like we're doing all the right things. It's frustrating. It's maddening. But all is not lost. In this section, we'll discuss some of the biological components of fat loss (or the lack thereof) and how we might be able to work with our bodies to get things going back in the right direction.

"MY MOM WaS FaT. MY DaD WaS FaT. I'M FaT."

It's a fact—many people have trouble losing weight and even more trouble keeping it off. But why is it so much more difficult for some people than others? Well, biology may play a role in that.

There is a fair amount of evidence that demonstrates that a portion of obesity can be inherited. That heritability, depending on the source, could account for anywhere between 30 percent and 70 percent of a person's obesity (168-170). One of those factors could cause problems with what are known as *uncoupling proteins*. These proteins are found in the mitochondria of your cells and are thought to be involved in thermogenesis (i.e., calorie burning) (169). When uncoupling proteins don't perform properly, they can mess with the body's ability to burn calories efficiently, which can obviously create issues with fat loss.

Another possible inherited issue leading to obesity is a mutation in any of several genes that regulate appetite, hormones, or the body's ability to burn calories (168-170). In particular, the genes that regulate leptin could cause major problems with weight gain and appetite control. Leptin is a hormone produced by the body's fat cells, and it basically tells your brain whether you need to eat. When leptin isn't functioning properly, or when the brain isn't receiving signals from leptin for some reason, the body assumes that you need food, and your appetite increases. Genetic factors that affect leptin seem to result in severe weight gain (168-170).

There are other genes that can affect fat regulation. A gene called FTO seems to be involved with satiety, so when there is a defect there, it can affect hunger levels and how much people eat as a result (171-

172). There are multiple other genes that work alone or with FTO to mess with the body's food intake regulation capabilities, and these all could have a hand in causing weight gain (168-172).

PERIMENOPAUSE AND MENOPAUSE: "I LOST WEIGHT EASILY BEFORE"

Menopause and hormonal issues were a popular subject on my little social media thread about weight-loss obstacles. And there does seem to be a relationship between aging, hormones, and fat gain. Women in general have a higher incidence of severe obesity across the globe than men (173). The loss of estrogen that comes with menopause and other diseases of the female reproductive system seems to cause an increase in fat, as well as a decrease in muscle mass. Therefore, while body weight might not change, body composition certainly will. Rising estrogen levels can dampen your appetite during the menstrual cycle and can lower cravings for sweet foods during those higher estrogen phases of the cycle (173), so it stands to reason that a loss of estrogen might increase appetite and cravings.

Remember the visceral fat we talked about earlier? Well, that can jump from about 5 percent to 8 percent of total body fat to 15 percent to 20 percent total body fat after menopause (174). This may be due to hormones or aging, or it may be a combination of the two. The majority of sources seem to think that overall body size is related more to age, while fat distribution is related to hormones, but the jury is still out on that (174). There is also some evidence that women who have had medically induced menopause (due to hysterectomy, for instance) had a higher risk of severe obesity than women whose menopause happened naturally (174).

Increases in androgen (the "male" hormone; we all have some male and female hormones inside us) and decreases in sex hormone–binding globulin, which is a hormone that binds some types of testosterone and some types of estrogen (among other hormones). When androgen testosterone levels are higher in women, it can result in weight gain (174). Basically, we have a situation in which there are higher androgen levels and lower hormones to bind them, which can be a recipe for weight gain.

Aging in general can also interfere with body mass, in that physical activity—both amount and intensity—seems to decrease with age (174-175). This means that fewer calories are burned, and that nothing will mitigate the loss of muscle mass that comes along with aging. We've seen the effects cardiovascular activity can have on visceral fat earlier in this book, and as we are now discovering, visceral fat seems to be a much bigger problem after menopause. A lack of physical exercise is a big deal.

Aging and hormonal fluctuations during menopause also interfere with sleep. Night sweats, mood swings, restless leg syndrome, awakening often throughout the night, waking up too early, and sleep apnea can all occur with menopause and perimenopause (175-176). With lack of sleep, the body cannot repair itself, appetite and cravings increase, physical activity tends to be reduced, and body fat tends to increase (175, 177).

The good news is that all is not lost for those who are going through menopause, or even for those who have a genetic predisposition for obesity. Menopausal weight gain and other symptoms can be treated with menopausal hormone therapy (MHT). There are actually a lot of benefits to estrogen therapy for menopause, including a lower risk of heart attack, a lower risk of death, improved bone strength, improved parameters on a lot of the issues that come along with menopause (sexual health, mood, etc.), general quality of life improvements, and more (175, 178). There are some risks that might come along with hormone therapy as well, though: There may be a slight increase in breast cancer risk and stroke risk, but transdermal versions of MHT may mitigate some of these risks. However, the current global consensus on the use of MHT is that the benefits outweigh the risks (178). It's worth discussing with your doctor.

That said, physical activity has been found to help reign in both menopausal (or age-related) (174-175) and in genetic (179-180) increases in fat. Increasing lean muscle and increasing caloric burn seem to go a long way in keeping fat at bay, even when the odds seem against you. So don't throw in the proverbial towel just because you think you're "too old." It may seem daunting to get on the exercise bandwagon when your energy levels are low and you feel like everything is working against you, but the odds are that it will work in your favor.

Burning off more calories than you take in is still needed for weight loss, even when there are biological factors in play.

Intensity, duration, and frequency of exercise all play a role in success, so make sure you stay consistent, move often, and challenge yourself. Current recommendations for people considered obese (about 30 lb overweight or more) are to work up to about 200 to 300 minutes per week, or about 30 to 45 minutes daily; some reports recommend 60 to 90 minutes daily (181-182). A higher-intensity training program could cut down on the amount of time needed to have the same effect (182).

Make no mistake—you'll still need to reign in your calorie intake. Burning off more calories than you take in is still needed for weight loss, even when there are biological factors in play. But physical exercise becomes more and more important the older you get.

When it comes down to it, much like dieting, the best exercise is the kind you are willing to do. So find a physical outlet that you can at least tolerate, if not fully enjoy, and make it happen on the regular. Your body will thank you for it.

"SOMETIMES IT FEELS LIKE MY BODY IS HAPPY AT 240 TO 260 POUNDS."

There are a few theories in scientific circles regarding the body wanting to remain at a certain weight. The most well-known is the *set point theory*, which states that the body perceives a specific weight range as where it needs to be, so it sends signals to eat and burn what is needed to stay within that range. Another theory is the *settling point theory*, in which the body settles at a weight based on the environment it is in. If a person is somewhere where food is good and plentiful and there isn't much need for movement, the body will settle at a higher level than it would if that person was in a place where food is scarce, or in which that person does very large amounts of physical activity on a regular basis. The settling point will change based on the requirements of that person's environment.

While these are not the only theories of the body's internal regulation of weight, they are the best known. And the fact of the matter is that there is no consensus or real proof of either one. There is not only evidence to support both theories (and several others), but plenty of evidence against the theories as well. And when it comes down to it, no one knows for sure if the body regulates its weight at all (186-187).

What we do know is that if there is a set point, settling point, or some other point, it can change based on consistent food intake and energy expenditure (i.e., exercise). If you find yourself at a weight loss plateau, there are several strategies you can use to try to break through it:

- *Increase your protein.* As we discussed earlier in this book, there is a certain thermic effect of protein, and protein can keep you feeling fuller longer. Including more protein in your diet might help give you an edge on burning a little more and eating a little less. It can also help fuel your muscles for those workouts, because you'll probably need to.

- *Move more.* Or at least move more intensely. Your body might have adapted to the pace at which you currently train, so you might need to move a little faster, run or walk on hills instead of flat ground, lift heavier weights, or increase the amount of time you do physical activity. If you're not weight training, add in some strength sessions. If you're not doing cardio, add some exercise to get your heart pumping. You can also start ramping up what is known as *NEAT*, or non-exercise activity thermogenesis. NEAT can really ramp up the number of calories you burn in a day (188), so you can do things like stand instead of sit, climb the escalator (or stairs) instead of riding it or taking the elevator, park a little further away from your destination than usual, carry your own bags at the market, and even fidget in your seat. The more you move, the better.

- *Eat more fiber.* An easy way to do this is to up your non-starchy veggie intake. Vegetables are not only full of fiber, but they are low in calories and dense in nutrients, so you can eat a lot of them and not really risk going overboard on your daily caloric needs. Fiber in general helps keep you feeling full (so you will likely eat less) and has many other health benefits to boot (189).

- *Drink more water.* Sometimes your body sends hunger signals when it's actually thirsty, so make sure you drink plenty of water to keep yourself hydrated. Water can also take up room in your stomach, leaving less room for food, so it keeps you from taking in more calories.

- *Check your sleep.* If you're not sleeping enough, your metabolism can actually drop, and sleep deprivation has been found to be a factor in weight gain (190). Most people need around seven to eight hours of quality shuteye per night, although there are variations in overall sleep requirements from person to person. We'll talk more about sleep hygiene later in this book, but if you try everything and can't figure out why you're still not sleeping right, you may want to talk to a qualified medical professional and figure out what's going on. And while you're at it . . .

- *Lower your stress levels.* High stress levels can not only interfere with sleep and exercise but can also trigger poor eating habits and behaviors (more on this later) (191). There are several ways to address stress (we'll talk about some of these later in this book). Find a method that works well for you and stick to it consistently. Stress is something that affects all of us; keeping it under control is extremely important.

- *Track your food.* It's possible that you're eating more (or a lot less) than you think you are. Tracking your food for a week or so can make you a lot more mindful of what's going into your body so that you can pinpoint issues you didn't realize were there.

If everything seems to be on target and your body fat still won't budge, you may want to talk to your doctor about having some tests done to ensure there's nothing awry with your hormones or anything else. Issues with the thyroid and other hormones can interfere with weight loss, and the right medication or medical plan can often set things right again.

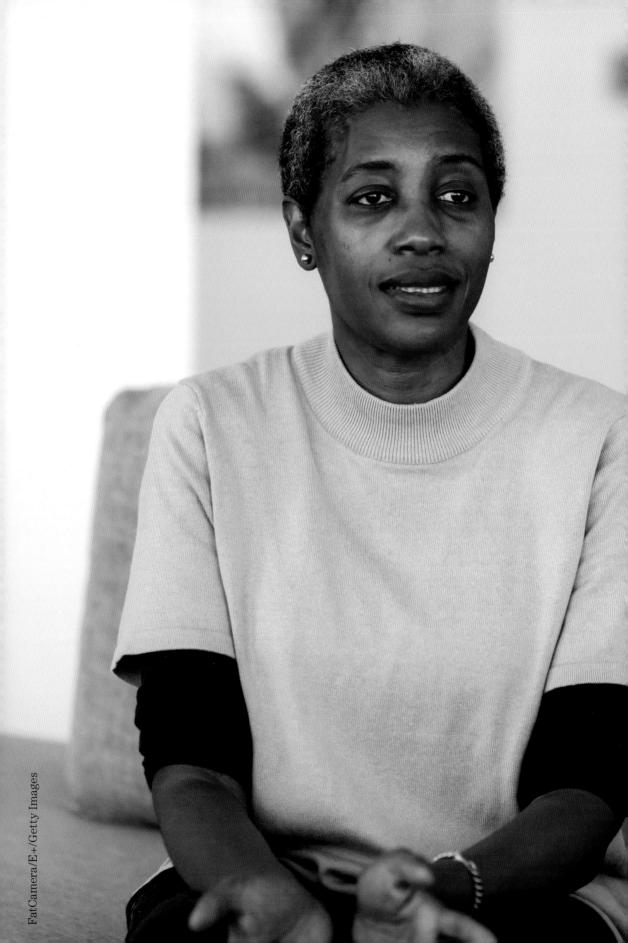

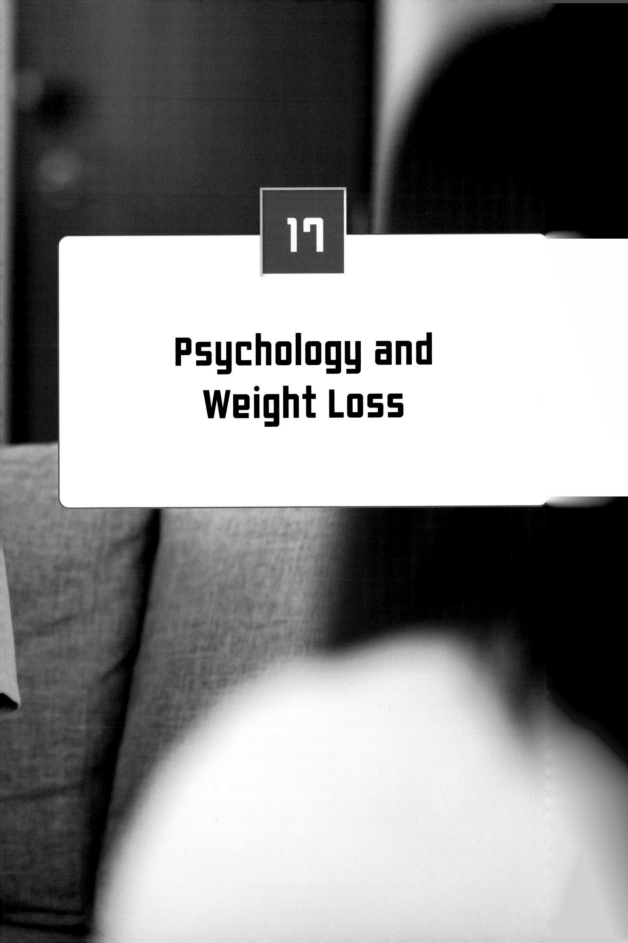

17

Psychology and Weight Loss

I got my master's degree in health psychology (with a concentration in food psychology) because humans have an incredibly mental and emotional relationship with food. That relationship is not always a healthy one and is not always logical. Food is social, food is love, food is comfort, and food is the answer we crave when we have no answers. And sometimes we need couples' counseling because our relationship with food can be kind of dysfunctional.

I had a client who had highly symptomatic diabetes and was sick and miserable in her body. She came to me desperate for help, but the very thought of changing even the smallest thing in her diet was so agonizing that it actually brought her to tears. This isn't unusual. Food is a security blanket that many people aren't willing to let go of, even when it's harming them. In this section, I'll discuss some of those psychological and emotional issues that commonly arise with eating and hopefully give some useful strategies on how to get back on track when everything feels like it's working against you.

> *"Figuring out how to beat sugar cravings . . . they keep me from making it to the final destination. I can exercise my way to where I want to be, but the sugar cravings keep me from maintaining."*

FIGHT THE CRAVINGS

I have a confession to make—I was a sugar-holic. I've never had an addiction in my life. I've never smoked anything, never tried one drug, and never even been drunk. But when it came to sugar, I was out of control. I'd eat it out of the bag with a spoon. If there was nothing sweet to eat in the house, I'd pour myself a glass of maple syrup. When I worked in corporate America (in another life, I was a computer consultant, believe it or not), I would go to the bulk candy store down the street from my office, buy up to 2 pounds of jelly beans in flavors no one liked but me (black licorice and cinnamon . . . mmmm) "for the office," and end up eating the whole bag in 30 minutes flat. Nothing was too sweet for me, and I could not get through the day without a massive dose of something sugary.

Whether sugar is addictive is a hot topic of debate in nutrition circles. In many scientific circles, the evidence surrounding sugar addiction is not found to be very convincing (183). Others, however, argue that the overlap between the brain's response to sugar and behaviors surrounding sugar indicate that sugar has addictive qualities (184). There doesn't seem to be a consensus in this area just yet.

As for my own experience, I can say that this was as addicted to anything as I've ever been (keeping in mind that I've never really been addicted to anything). I am certainly not going to compare it to street drugs, but for me it was a compulsion, and it was a beast to kick the habit. Whether or not there is any validity to the sugar-as-addiction theory, what I do know is that it's a monster many people wrestle with. There isn't much science on the best way to quit the sugar habit. I can tell you what worked for me in this case, and hopefully you'll find something helpful in that.

I got to the point where I realized that my need for sugar was kind of controlling my life in some ways, and I did not like that feeling at all. So I finally decided I'd had enough and set my mind to do something about it. I'd made feeble attempts to quit sugar in the past, but the fact of the matter was that I wasn't quite ready to really quit yet. And unless you are truly ready to make change happen, chances are that change ain't gonna happen. But I was finally ready and could accept the discomfort that I knew would come along with trying to get something that I enjoyed so much out of my life for good.

The first thing I realized was that I needed to get sugar, in all its forms, out of my house. I knew if they were around, I'd eat them, so I had to get rid of them. I removed bags of sugar (a bummer, since I love to bake), bottles of syrup, and any other sugar-based items I happened to have in my possession.

The next thing I decided to try to do was replace sugar with dried fruit. In my mind, I couldn't overeat dried fruit because if you overeat dried fruit you end up with a stomachache. Unfortunately, what happened was that I got immune to the stomachache and developed some sort of weird superpower in which I was able to consume huge amounts of dried fruit at once. Clearly dried fruit wasn't going to be my salvation, so I had to put the kibosh on that.

I finally settled on allowing myself three to four servings of fresh fruit per day. Other than that, I was not allowed to have any added sugars or sugary foods. I don't like to make this comparison, as I don't think the two substances are similar at all. But I liken it to this: You can't give a drug addict a little bit of their vice in order to help wean them off. And that's how it was for me—I knew I couldn't have a little bit of sugar, or it would turn into a whole lot of sugar, and the cycle would begin again.

For the first several days, it was *hard*. I had to basically sit on my hands to keep myself from going out and buying sugar, and I had kind of a mild version of the shakes for a day or two. I'm not gonna lie—it was miserable.

But a few weeks in, something interesting happened—I stopped really craving sugar. I didn't feel like I needed something sweet after meals, and I wasn't clamoring for candy. I was perfectly satisfied with the fresh fruit allotment for the day, and I wasn't consumed with thoughts of jelly beans. I didn't proclaim myself yet cured of my sugar cravings, but there was an obvious big change happening.

About four months in, I decided to allow myself to have dessert at a restaurant. Normally, I'd want my dessert and everyone else's, too. But now I found that not only was my dessert not as good as it looked, but it was actually too sweet for me. That was shocking. I had never had the experience before of something being too sweet for me. I used to be able to eat frosting out of the can with a spoon—now it kind of made my teeth itch; it was so sweet. I just didn't enjoy dessert like I used to, and I was fine having a bite or two and calling it a day. That was a huge victory.

That was in 2010. Ten years later, I'm still able to manage my sugar intake very well. I can have a bite of dessert and be completely satisfied with that, and jelly beans are a thing of my past. My only real kryptonite is when I make my chocolate crisp rice treats during the winter holidays—I can eat a whole pan of that stuff if I'm not careful. But for the most part, kicking the sugar habit has been a major victory for me.

That said, some people will never be able to let dessert be part of their lives again—everyone is different. The main thing I absolutely recommend, though, is to eliminate sugar completely until your cravings go away completely, and then decide for yourself if you're able to handle small amounts of the stuff again without going overboard. If you end up going back to your old habits, you'll probably have to repeat this process to break the cycle and keep sugary snacks a distant memory.

There is a possibility, I suppose, that your cravings will never completely go away, so it may end up being a constant state of willpower; everyone's body is different. However, most people (in my experience) who have gone this route have had good success, and I've yet to meet anyone who never lost their cravings.

"Keeping it up: I can exercise and diet for about three months, and then it starts to fall apart. It feels like a drug addiction. I just end up eating candy and not controlling portions the way I need to. And then I end up not exercising for a week here and there 'cause I don't feel well, or something physical feels less than perfect . . ."

"Not getting down on myself for small backslides."

"Depression. Obstacles in life. Emotional eating. Portion control. Unintentional sabotagers. The [all-or-nothing] (if you get a flat tire) mentality. I could go on."

"Wine and fattening foods with family and friends on the weekends. When I decide to lose some weight, I have to get away from everyone!"

"Here's a fun one—feeling like you deserve what you want, you've earned it!! Cue wine and Oreos!"

EMOTIONAL EATING

Issues surrounding emotional eating and self-sabotage were by far the most common comments that came up in my social media request. Emotional eating is something we've all struggled with from time to time, and it's hard to make sense of it sometimes, since it's not a rational beast.

A basic definition of *emotional eating* is spontaneous, non-hunger-based eating that is triggered by some sort of emotion, such as stress, depression, boredom, panic, anxiety, social situations, and even joy and celebrations. Emotional eating is often compared to binge eating, but there is a difference between the two; that difference is essentially the quantity of the foods being eaten. While emotional eating might be something like tearing into a pint of ice cream after a breakup, binge eating is rapidly consuming huge amounts of food to the point where you are phenomenally overstuffed. A binge-eating session might include hiding food or making sure binging sessions happen when you are alone (192). While emotional eating and binge eating aren't the same thing, they can be intertwined—emotional eating may lead to binge eating, or it may be part of an existing binge-eating disorder.

Causes For Emotional Eating

There is a reason why emotional eating feels good in the moment—eating kind of forces your body to relax, at least temporarily. Your body does not digest well when you're upset, so your parasympathetic nervous system kicks in and causes a "rest and digest" condition, so you'll often calm down a bit while you're eating (193). For some people, eating a lot of really tasty but not-so-healthy food (cake, candy, anything with a name ending in *-itos*, etc.) triggers reactions in the body that tell the brain that it needs food and dampens the reactions that tell the body to control the need for food (194-197). For these people, the brain always senses that it's starving, even when the body has consumed more than enough energy. This is a condition known as *leptin resistance*.

Most of us live in a high-stress world (whether it is of our own making or not), and for those of us who are susceptible to it, stress exacerbates leptin resistance. Guess what else contributes to stress? That's right—failed dieting (196). So there ends up being this vicious cycle: A person tries a diet, gets frustrated, gets off the diet, gets stressed out due to

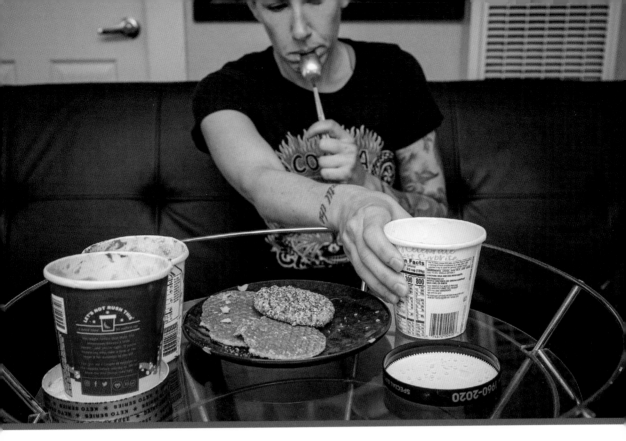

the diet not working, eats in response to the stress, and ends up back at square one. The result is an inability to decipher real hunger signals, so eating happens regardless of whether the person is hungry or not.

Another thing that can contribute to emotional eating is a woman's monthly cycle. Women appear to binge eat the most during periods of negative emotions, which are generally worst during the mid-luteal and premenstrual phases of their cycles (198). During this time, fluctuations in the levels of hormones called *estradiol* and *progesterone* interact to contribute to emotional-eating tendencies. Interestingly, this also seems to go hand in hand with the highest concerns about body weight (198). So a woman will feel the need to eat in response to negative feelings and then will start to become worried about the effects of that eating on her physique.

The tendency to emotionally eat during the menstrual cycle seems to be stronger in women who have a clinical history of binge eating, so we can again see that relationship between emotional eating and binge eating (198). They aren't the same, but they often appear together.

For many people, emotional eating starts in childhood (199). It may be that a parental figure exhibits dysfunctional eating patterns that the child emulates, or it may be that the parent enforces a dysfunctional eating pattern in the child that overrides hunger sensations (i.e., phrases like "clean your plate!" or giving junk foods to pacify a distraught child, etc.).

Emotional eating seems to be more prevalent in girls and women and may also be more prevalent in LGBTQ+ individuals (200). There is also a possible genetic susceptibility to those who emotionally eat, and this may be visible in childhood (201-202). As we have seen before, though, a genetic predisposition to dysfunctional eating makes things more difficult but is not a complete roadblock to fat loss success. We'll discuss some solutions a bit later in this section.

There are other causes of emotional eating. One of those is an emotional blockage—the inability to express or identify one's feelings (203). Not being able to express oneself can lead to feelings of frustration, depression, and isolation, and often things become internalized. This, of course, leads to more stress, and we saw earlier how stress can cause emotional eating. In this case, the person is essentially "eating their feelings."

Another cause is almost the opposite—people who have difficulty controlling or managing their emotions can also end up lashing out and becoming very frustrated, with the same stress pattern appearing (203). Either one of these emotional traits may have been learned in childhood or may have developed over time.

Post-traumatic stress disorder (PTSD) from abusive or traumatic experiences in childhood or adulthood can wreak havoc on the body's ability to regulate hunger signals (203). Normally, the body responds to stress by decreasing appetite (because the body needs to "rest and digest," shutting down the appetite until everything calms down). However, in some cases of PTSD, appetite signals get mixed up, and the opposite happens—the stress causes the body to think it needs to eat (which, as we discussed earlier, will probably force it to calm down a bit).

WHAT DO I DO ABOUT IT?

Emotional eating can make us feel helpless, can make us feel awful about ourselves, and can send us into a tailspin of unhealthy habits.

Fortunately, there are strategies to help you get beyond this issue and back on track.

First of all, it's important to realize that emotional eating is only a problem if it's a chronic issue. If you had a bad day and ate a sleeve of Oreos once, that doesn't necessarily constitute a problem. If you do something like that every time you're feeling bored, stressed, sad, or angry, and it's become a regular thing that derails your health and happiness, then the emotional eating has become a pattern and needs to be dealt with.

Know Your Triggers

The first strategy to use when dealing with emotional eating is figuring out what triggers you. It may not be obvious at first, so one thing I recommend to everyone is to keep a food log for at least a week. It doesn't have to be forever—this is just to understand unhealthy patterns so that we can break them. Your food diary might look something like this:

Time of Day	Food Type and Quantity	Was I Hungry?	What Was My Mood When I Ate?
12:30 p.m.	1 family pack of tortilla chips	No	I was feeling lonely.
3:24 p.m.	1 cup baby carrots	Yes	I felt hungry and carrots always help me feel fuller.
5:13 p.m.	2 lb jelly beans	No	I was watching TV and needed to munch on something. Before I knew it, all the jelly beans were gone.

In this log, we see that this person's triggers might be feeling sad or lonely, and feeling bored or having a mindless eating pattern when watching TV—if the pattern continues every time they experience these emotions, this can be confirmed. We could discover, upon logging for a longer time, that this person craves crunchy and salty foods when feeling sad or lonely and sweet foods when watching TV. Once you know your triggers and how you respond to them, you can start to address those situations directly.

Become Mindful

When you eat based on your emotions, you are often on autopilot. As soon as you feel sad, stressed, bored, or anxious emotion, you reach for all the snacks, and you don't really think about it much. Now is the time to start thinking about it. Becoming aware of what and why you are eating in the moment can put a jolt in your usual automatic response to pacify an emotion with food (204). When you find yourself reaching for food in the wake of a triggering situation, try first asking yourself the following questions:

- Am I *really* hungry right now, or am I just eating to eat?
- Will this food solve my problem?
- Will this food make me feel better right now?
- Will this food make me feel better in one hour?
- What is something else I can do right now to address my problem?

Taking the time to ask yourself these questions can pull you out of autopilot and make you consider your actions before you go back to old habits. You can then take one of the following additional steps.

Be Prepared

When you are not in a trigger situation, take some time to make a list of nonfood-related things you can do to help yourself get through a rough spot. You might, for instance, choose to "take a walk," which is an awesome idea. But what if it's raining, or what if it's midnight? That's why having a few options that cover all your bases is a good idea. Your list, then, might look like this:

> **Stuff to Do When I Feel Stressed**
> Take a walk
> Call Tracy, Stu, Ed, or Mandy
> Do a puzzle
> Punch a punching bag or pillow
> Take a warm bath
> Listen to a guided meditation

This list now includes things you can do regardless of the time or weather. Note that the list has more than one person for calling just in case some of those people aren't available. It is a good idea to let the people on your call list know that you might call them during trigger times to help talk you down from an emotional eating situation. That way, they can be better prepared to help you when needed.

Now that you have your list, keep it with you! Put a copy on your fridge, put a copy in your wallet, paste a copy to your bathroom mirror, or anywhere you can easily see it and be reminded of it no matter where you happen to be. Pick something feasible on the list and do it—don't stop and think about it too much. Get your brain off food as quickly as you can and redirect to another activity.

Learn Coping Skills

Learning to regulate and respond appropriately to emotions can be an important step in removing the need for food-soothing. If you are open to it, this may be best achieved through standard or enhanced behavioral therapy (205), or even through a support group. A quick Internet search for "emotional eating support group" pulls up a host of different groups, both virtual and in-person, that you might find useful to help learn how to express your emotions healthfully.

Live in the Present

We often berate ourselves for having eaten something we think we shouldn't have and label ourselves "bad" or "failure" as a result. This often makes people think, "Well, I screwed that up. Might as well just call it quits now." It is so tempting to let one setback negate all your efforts. But remember this: You cannot change what you have already done. You can only change the present. Quitting everything obviously isn't going to improve your situation, so ask yourself this:

What is one thing I can do to change the present?

It is possible that you tried to do too much at once. In that case, scale it back and try making incremental small changes (more on this later). Or perhaps you tried to push yourself to change something you weren't ready to change yet. In that case, give that one thing a rest and concentrate on making positive changes elsewhere. You don't have to be perfect—you just have to be headed in the right direction. Every small step makes a difference. I know it's hard to sometimes see that in the moment, but taking a step back and getting some perspective can help. In any event, even though it's easy to just say "to hell with it" and go back to your old ways, try not to let yourself take the easy way out. Stop beating yourself up, take some time, take a breath, clear your mind, and think about one small way you can do things better right now.

Try Slowing Down Your Eating

It takes your body a while to figure out that you're full, so don't outpace it. Try taking twice as long to eat as usual. Savor every bite; think about how it tastes, what the texture is like, how it makes you feel when you eat it—that sort of thing. This is one way to remain mindful while you eat so that you don't end up halfway through a bag of chips before you realize what you've done.

Delay Gratification

When you're tempted to emotionally eat, try delaying your access to food, even if it's just for a few minutes. The longer you can delay access, the better. But it might just be five minutes at first. Still, that 5 minutes (or 20 minutes, or whatever you can manage) does a whole lot: It can give you more of a sense of control of what and when you are eating, and it gives you time to ask yourself those mindfulness questions I mentioned earlier. Plus, by the time your food delay has passed, your craving might have passed, too.

Make a Plan

Emotional eating doesn't just happen when you're feeling bad or bored. It also happens during social occasions and when you want to celebrate yourself or have an "I earned this" moment. If you overdo it during social events and outings, make a plan for those times. At restaurants, have the waitstaff pack up half of your food before bringing it to the table so you don't munch on food because it's in front of you (and then you'll have your lunch for the next day—bonus!) Get appetizer portions instead of full portions, or share a full meal with a dining partner or share a few appetizers. If you want to go whole hog, adjust what you're eating for the rest of the day so that you have room to indulge a little in the evening. If alcohol is your nemesis, get one drink and make it last the entire evening. With your drink, get a huge glass of water; with every sip of your drink, have a big gulp of water. That way, you'll still get to drink your alcohol, but you won't down glass after glass, and the water is a method of staying mindful of your intake.

Find ways to celebrate yourself that have nothing to do with food—give yourself a mini-vacation (or a maxi-vacation if you can!), a spa day, or an outing to somewhere interesting, maybe something at the store you've been eyeing.

Social Networks as a Secret Weapon

"Outside (negative) influences—family not into it, having their bad food in the house & their lack of discipline/caring, same at work with vendors bringing in sweets[. . .] to the office & invites to happy hour[. . . .]"

Have you ever been out with a group of friends and ate all kinds of things you didn't intend to eat just because everyone else was? Or have you ever been in a relationship in which you gained weight because your partner loves snack foods, which are now always in the house and tempting you like crazy? Yep. Fat loss has a major social factor.

A lot of outside influences can affect your drive to snack. Perhaps your family simply doesn't want to eat what you're eating, and if you're the family chef, now you have to make two or more meals every time you cook. Maybe you have a coworker who loves to bring in cookies and candy, or someone in your house leaves bags of chips everywhere and isn't willing to stop. Then there's the happy hour invites, the office parties, the dinners out with friends who order all the appetizers for the table to share . . . well, it's hard to resist, isn't it?

I have a client who has gained and lost the same 40 pounds over and over and over again over the years. She knows what she needs to do and sincerely wants to lose the fat. However, her husband prefers her to be bigger and really gets on her case when she loses fat. This is a major factor in her never being able to stick with a plan for much longer than a year. It's really hard to try to get healthy when the person you live with fights you every step of the way.

A supportive social network has been proven over and over to significantly improve your chances of losing fat and maintaining that loss. A lot of people seem to want to keep their fitness journeys a secret from their friends and family. If you are one of them, I don't doubt that you have very valid reasons for it. However, I'd like to recommend that you tell the people you hang out with the most, especially if you eat with these people. Tell them what you're trying to achieve. Ask that they help respect your choices as you reach for your goals. Most of the time, people will be more than willing to cheer you on and help you out; sometimes, you'll even inspire them to join you!

However, there are always those that remain unsupportive. It's easy enough to say that you shouldn't eat with those people, but that isn't always feasible (like in the case of my client and her husband). In that case, it will definitely be much harder for you to stay on track. However, it can be done. Exercising your willpower is part of it—you have to figure out a way to avoid the temptation to overeat while around these unsupportive people. I realize this is easier said than done; but it can be done. Say "no" to the temptations at the office; make your own food at home. I completely understand that this can be very difficult and forces you to do more work; unfortunately, it's a necessary obstacle you'll need to tackle in order to achieve your goals.

In addition, I recommend finding a supportive group of people outside of the unsupportive relationship (or relationships). You may find a walking group in your area or a great group of people at the gym. There might be a healthy eating group in your area or maybe a group of people who are trying to lose fat healthfully. Websites such as Meetup, SparkPeople, WeightLossBuddy, and others can be good places to look for supportive people who are on your same wavelength. You can also join Internet support groups (there are several on social media sites such as Facebook) if needed, as they can be extremely helpful and motivating for many people. While you may not be getting the backup you need at home or within your personal circle, you can still get the support you need outside of that. And that can make all the difference in the world.

avoid Self-Sabotage

"All these different diet programs have left me with a list of 'rules' about food in my head—some of which actually contradict each other. That, plus the all-or-nothing restrict/binge cycle that dieting has created in my head means that I'm either super strict and adhering to all these different rules, or I'm all "screw the rules" and eating everything that's not nailed down. Then, because I've assigned all these value judgements to food because of those rules (good foods vs. bad foods), I wind up assigning those same value judgements to myself based on how I'm eating—which leads down a whole other road with emotional eating and all that jazz. And in spite of being able to identify all these issues with my rational mind, I still struggle with all of it. And that's the long and (not so) short of it."

"Media/society shaming me. Can't do what you need to do when [there are] constant reminders that you aren't good enough create shame spirals."

"I feel like a failure. I haven't done what I planned this week, and I feel like all my hard work is ruined now. I'm ready to quit again. I just want to eat everything in sight and call it a day."

Self-sabotage is a nasty beast. For many, it's spurned by a need for perfection, and anything deemed less than perfect becomes failure. For others, it's a sense of hopelessness when results don't come quickly enough or have backtracked in some way. Some people set for themselves very high standards that they aren't quite able to meet, and some people feel that they are failures unless they look a certain way, act a certain way, or are perceived by others a certain way. Sometimes it's a fear of the unknown or a fear of change. Regardless of what fuels the fire, the thing that most self-destructive behaviors stem from is a feeling of shame (208). When people don't meet the goals that they set for themselves, they feel ashamed or guilty. They become extremely self-critical, labeling themselves as failures, as inadequate, as inferior, as unworthy, as "bad," or a host of other not-so-nice things. They may feel depressed, rejected, isolated, unwanted, or unloved. They try to moderate those feelings, which, of course, are extremely uncomfortable feelings to have, by exhibiting self-destructive behaviors. Those behaviors could manifest as binge eating, anorexia, substance abuse, or other dangerous endeavors.

Some people, consciously or not, find a sort of comfort in remaining overweight. In a way, it is a protective blanket that keeps them from having to get more involved in life (which can be really scary for some people). It's a good excuse to explain why certain things aren't working out, and it's a "get out of jail free" card from being told how to eat and move. Or perhaps if they're not *trying* to lose weight, then that means they don't actually *have* to lose weight. Maybe they think that with extra weight, people don't see them as a threat, so they feel more socially accepted.

If you self-sabotage, it's important to figure out what's behind your actions. You may need help doing this, so speaking to a qualified professional could help to get to the bottom of what's stopping your progress. There are, however, some tactics you can try on your own to try to get out of a destructive cycle.

Make Small Goals for Yourself

Don't aim for anything huge. Aim for something extremely manageable that you can do in the next week or two. Give yourself regular goals like this:

Week 1: Take a walk after work.
Week 2: Don't get fast food.
Week 3: Drink 8 ounces of water with every meal.

Don't set goals too far in advance (i.e., don't set week 3's goals before you've finished week 1), and make sure you set goals that are both feasible and relatively easy for you to achieve. Reward yourself with something nonfood-related that makes you feel good every time you hit a goal. (More on goal setting later in this book.) Setting a goal gives you something manageable to aim for, and reaching goals gives us a little dopamine hit (the "feel good" chemicals in the brain), so it motivates us to keep doing good for ourselves.

Change Your Perspective

It's easy to berate yourself over the things you think you've done wrong. But the chances are that doing that is overshadowing your ability to see everything you've been doing right. Make a physical list of things you've been doing well, things that are good about you, and things that are good in your life. If you need to, enlist the help of a supportive friend to help you make your list. Put that list somewhere very visible and refer to it often. Add to it whenever you can—once a week or more if possible. Even the smallest things ("I rescued a spider from my bathroom and put it safely outside"; "I make really good soup.") make a difference. Don't be modest. Now is the time to make the good stuff loudest.

Do One Thing Every Day to Practice Self-Care

This can be anything nondestructive that makes you feel good, from listening to a song you love to slowing way down while you eat so you can actually enjoy your food.

Punch Something

When I have stressed-out clients come in, I hand them a club and something to hit and let them have at it. They wail on punching bags, smack chains repeatedly into the ground, and just get their anger out. I even had shirts made up for my business that say, "I feel better when I hit things." Because you know what? Sometimes you just need to hit something. Some people like to scream at the top of their lungs. Some people like to write down all of their negative thoughts and burn them in the fireplace. It doesn't matter as long as it works for you. Get your frustration out in a safe and nondestructive way. That way you can get into a place where frustration isn't consuming you, and you can perhaps take a step back to try to get some perspective. Ask yourself: Is what I'm telling myself really true? Are things really as bad as I'm making them out to be? Are my expectations of myself realistic? Chances are, you'll be able to see that you can change the myths you've been feeding yourself and start to forgive yourself (or whoever needs forgiving) and start to turn things around for the better. If you find this impossible, getting qualified outside help might be worth looking into.

Pay Attention

Understand that you're probably not going to completely reverse long-held beliefs about yourself or the urge to beat yourself up. But you can stop feeding the dragon. Identify when you're starting to spiral and don't let it get worse. Talk to supportive people when necessary, get out in nature, or do whatever you need to do to be kind to yourself and get into a better headspace.

I don't claim to have all the solutions—I just have a few ideas that have worked for my clients and myself in the past. Hopefully, you'll find some of them helpful, or you'll find another way that works for you to get back to a healthy place.

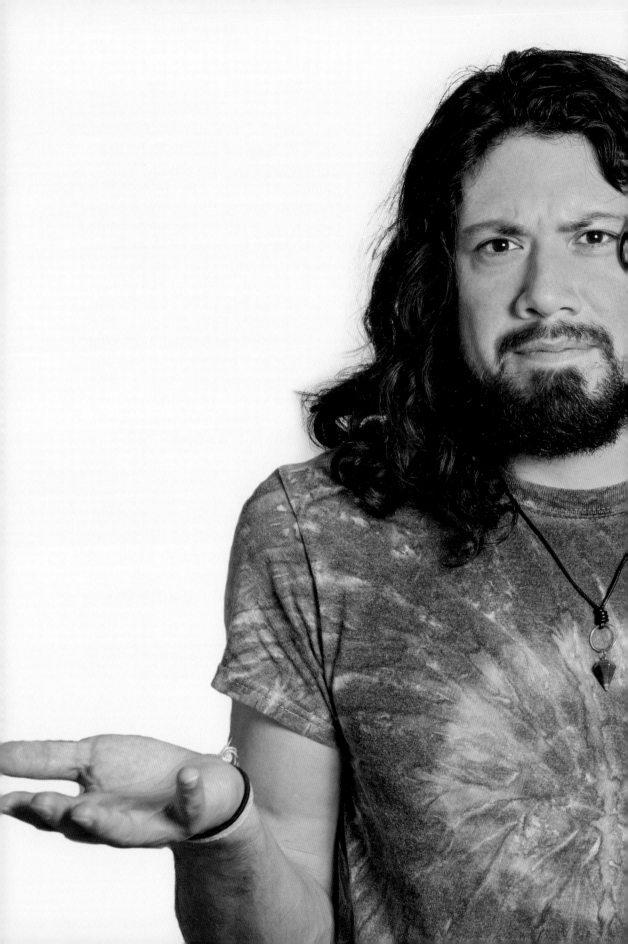

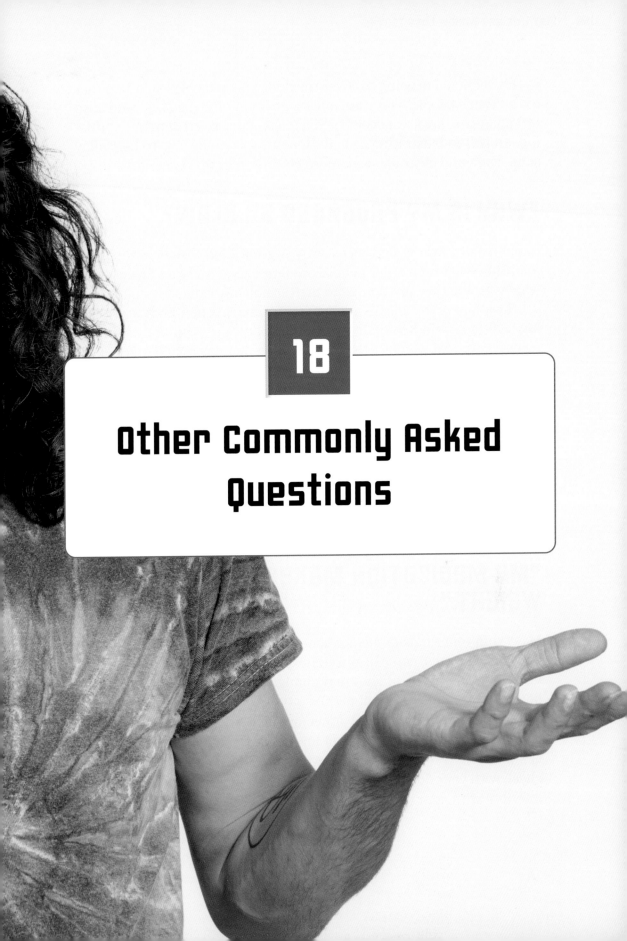

18

Other Commonly Asked Questions

In this section, I'm going to cover the odds and ends of weight loss that often stymie people. These are questions I hear often and that were also brought up on my great social media quest. Fat loss is complex, confusing, and often frustrating as hell. Hopefully, I will be able to help allay some fears and clear up some more confusion in this part of the book.

"WHY IS MY PROGRESS SO SLOW?"

Rapid weight loss is not necessarily a great idea. I understand how tempting it is to see other people's weight loss success and want to do whatever it is they are doing, no matter how unrealistic it might be. I get the allure of the ads promising you an amazing new body and glowing health. Weight loss reality shows don't become popular by showing healthy, gradual weight loss; they become popular by making people puke, severely restricting the contestants' diets, and beating the living garbage out of them until the contestants lose tremendous amounts of weight and look amazing and weep tears of joy (and, in the vast majority of cases, gain the weight back not long after the show ends).

I don't mean to be redundant, but I'm going to be. When you look at programs that make big, lofty promises, ask yourself: Can I do this forever? Be honest. If the answer is no, save your money no matter how great the results seem to be. A temporary program (or a program you stick to temporarily) will not give you lasting fat loss.

"MY MEDICATION MAKES ME GAIN WEIGHT."

Many different kinds of medications, including many antidepressants and steroid drugs, can cause weight gain due to fluid imbalances and changes in metabolism. They may change the distribution of fat in your body or may change your appetite so that you end up eating more.

Talk to your doctor about other options that may not have these kinds of side effects. If this is not an option (managing your condition is important, too), there are other things you can try (make sure you check with your doctor to make sure doing some of these things won't interfere with your medication):

- Cutting down on salt can help reduce water weight gain. Check food labels for added sodium in packaged foods and go for low-sodium or no-sodium options.
- Eat more lean protein and fiber to keep you feeling fuller for longer, and hopefully mitigate appetite changes. When you need to snack, snack on low-calorie, nutrient-dense foods like cut-up veggies. They may not be what you're craving, but they'll help fill you up.
- Keep exercising! Physical activity helps with mood and burns calories, so don't leave it to the wayside.
- Make sure you pay attention to your sleep quality—more on sleep later.

Really, all the tips mentioned in this book are valid for trying to lose weight gained through medicine, but it may be a bit more challenging. Don't despair, though—it's still quite possible to keep things under control.

TEMPTATION FOODS

"Time, money, not being the shopper or cook so [there is] less control over options . . ."

"Eating late [at] night and eating sweets"

"Eating my kids' food."

I'm going to tell you something that you're not going to want to hear, so I apologize in advance. If there are temptation foods in the house, you pretty much have two choices: Get them out or get them somewhere that you can't access them. Talk to your family or housemates about not having the foods that derail you in the house anymore. If they are OK with it, start immediately: Throw them out, donate them to a shelter, give them to a neighbor—just get them out of the house as soon as possible. Now it's on you to make sure they don't come back.

If the people you share your home with aren't down for getting rid of the stuff, work with them to make the snacky foods inaccessible to you. Hide it somewhere, lock it up—do whatever is needed to keep them out of your hands. If the food isn't around for you to eat, you won't binge on it. Much like the sugar conundrum, eventually you'll lose the urge to grab the munchy stuff. Until that happens, it just shouldn't be an option.

You may not be the shopper or the cook, but you can talk to the shopper (or the cook) and talk about your goals and what you'd like at the store. If they are supportive, you can put together grocery lists together and look up healthier recipes you both might like. If they aren't so supportive, well, we'll discuss that later in this book.

Eating healthy doesn't have to break the bank. Did you know that a lot of the bigger dollar-type stores often sell produce, as well as things like whole-grain bread, brown rice, and quinoa? If you live in an area with Asian or Mexican grocery stores, produce is often cheaper there as well. There are even services that aim to reduce food waste by selling "ugly" fruits and veggies (such as Imperfect Foods). Others sell healthy products that are near the end of their shelf life or are otherwise perfectly good but not likely to be sold in markets (such as FlashFood) at a big discount. If you have a green thumb, you can also try doing a garden share, which is where you grow your own produce and share your bounty with other gardeners in your area. You'll end up with a lot of great, super-fresh foods and maybe even a new friend or two. There are options out there—you just have to look for them!

KICK-STARTING

> *"I am going to cut out dairy and meat and gluten and sugar and joy for a few weeks to kick-start my body. Then I'll get on a good plan."*

A lot of my clients come to me telling me that they're going to temporarily cut out all kinds of things from their diet such as beans, wheat, fruits, certain vegetables, and so on in order to "kick-start" their plan and then slowly add them back in as the diet goes on. Basically, all this kick-starting is doing is putting you on a temporary extreme weight loss plan. And when it comes down to it, that is a pretty ineffective strategy.

Your body isn't going to think, "Oh, she didn't eat _____ for two weeks, so I'll just keep that weight loss going when she puts those foods back!" Basically, kick-starts work the same way all other diets do, which we know is—say it with me—caloric deficit.

COPYCATTING

"My neighbor went on X diet and they feel amazing now. Their joints don't hurt and their energy is so much higher. So I am going to try X diet, too!"

If you have a lot of weight to lose and you lose even some of it, you'll likely feel better. It isn't necessarily because your diet is so miraculous, but rather that you have a lowered risk of the complications that obesity causes and less pressure on your joints. You'll likely have more energy due to being able to move a little better and perhaps due to being happier with what you see in the mirror. So most people on most diets will claim that they feel healthier and have less pain. Once again, find what works for *you*. Chances are that you'll end up feeling a whole lot better, too.

VEGGIE HATERS

A lot of people are adverse to vegetables. There are potential solutions to this that you can try:

It Might Be How They're Cooked

I knew someone who hated cauliflower until they tried it roasted, and suddenly it was a whole new world. I had no idea I liked Brussels sprouts until I roasted them to the right consistency. It may be that you just have not had a vegetable cooked the right way. Try roasting, broiling, sautéing, air-frying, or barbequing veggies; look up interesting recipes that use them—give them a few chances before you cut them from your list. You might surprise yourself.

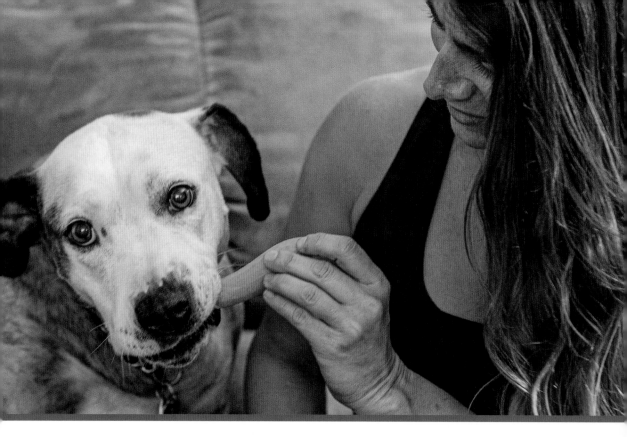

It Might Be How They're Cut

I know someone else who hates mushrooms—that is, unless they're cut really small. Then it's no big deal. Some people are texture people and having big chunks of veggies isn't their thing. Try different kinds of chopping methods, spiralizing, and so on, and see if that changes your mind.

You Might Need to Disguise Them

I have a secret: Sometimes I mix red lentils in with pasta sauce. You never know they're there, and they add a protein-and-nutrient kick. Parents have successfully been pureeing veggies into their kids' food for ages—give it a shot with your own. You might be surprised! Cauliflower is an easy one because it's pretty neutral and blends in with most other foods. Try pureeing it and mixing it in with pasta, mashed potatoes, or rice. You can puree red, orange, or yellow veggies and throw them in marinara sauce, and you can try mixing pureed greens into meatballs (or non-meatballs if you don't eat meat). Also, remember that many herbs also count as green veggies, so season your food well!

Try Pesto

Pesto is really a different way of sneaking pureed veggies into food. You can use almost any kind of green vegetable, plus garlic, salt, a little olive oil. Throw it on pasta or use it wherever you like pesto.

There are a ton of different vegetables out there. Make it a point every week to test out one you've never tried before and see how it goes. Maybe you'll get a new favorite!

Try a Green Drink

You might just need to drink your veggies if nothing else works. Mix greens into a smoothie or a protein shake, or get a protein shake that has veggies mixed into the ingredients (some of the "total meal" shakes have lots of veggies in them—read the ingredients and check). There are also greens powders that you can try. They probably won't taste great to you (most of them taste . . . well . . . green), but you can choke them down and get them out of the way. Some greens powders have flavor added to them, which might help make them a little more palatable for you. But anyway, just know that you have options. Like anything else, you just have to figure out what will work for you.

HEALTHY DOES NOT EQUAL LOWER CALORIES

I hear this one a lot, and the solution is to usually track everything they eat (there are plenty of free apps for this) for a week or two. If you've been recording everything you eat and still don't understand what's wrong, you may need to start weighing your food rather than just measuring it. Think about it this way: If you measure a cup of flour, and then measure another cup of flour but really pack it down, then you're going to end up with a whole lot more flour in the packed cup, right? And that can add up to considerably more calories than you thought you were eating. Weighing food can be an extremely useful tool if you really want to be as accurate as possible about how many calories per day you're actually eating.

What people often end up seeing is that even if what they're consuming is full of healthy ingredients, they're actually eating more calories than they're burning off. It pays to check yourself now and then—you might be surprised at what you find out.

One caveat is that if you're someone who is prone to eating disorders or becoming obsessive about food, weighing and measuring your food may not be the best avenue for you, and that might trigger problematic behaviors and attitudes toward food. There are other ways to estimate what portion sizes should look like. Try some of the following:

- *Hand measurements:* You can use your hand to figure out basic portion sizes. Meats and fish would be about the size of your palm. One thumb would be about the size of a serving of fats. Your fist would be about the size of a serving of grains or fruits. Two cupped hands would be about a serving of veggies.

- *Salad plates:* Subbing a salad plate for a dinner plate is an easy way to cut down portion sizes easily without thinking too much about it if you're not going back for seconds and thirds.

- *Plate portions:* Fill about half of your plate with veggies (not fried or doused in high-calorie sauces or oil, of course). Divide the other half into half-protein and half-whole grains.

Macro

Macro, short for *macronutrients*, is a term that basically encompasses the three big nutrients you eat every day: proteins, carbs, and fats. Counting macros is pretty much just another way of counting calories—if you get w grams of protein, x grams of carbs, and y grams of fat, you'll be getting z calories for the day. One advantage counting macros has is that it keeps you aware of how much of each macro you're eating every day. As a result, you might find that you're really low in protein, or perhaps you're super high in fat. As you discover a better dietary balance, you might feel better and perform better than you did before.

So, to answer the question: Do I need to count macros? No, of course not. It is one tool of many that can help you learn proper portion sizes and nutrient intake. If it works for you, absolutely do it. If it doesn't, there are plenty of other ways.

MEAL PLANS

Meal plans seem like a great idea; they take the guesswork out of food preparation, and you don't have to think so much about what you're going to eat. The downside is that people tend to get bored with meal plans, and they don't transfer well to social situations (this is why I'll generally say no when people ask me if I will write them a meal plan). So yeah, you *could* do a meal plan, but is that how you want to eat forever?

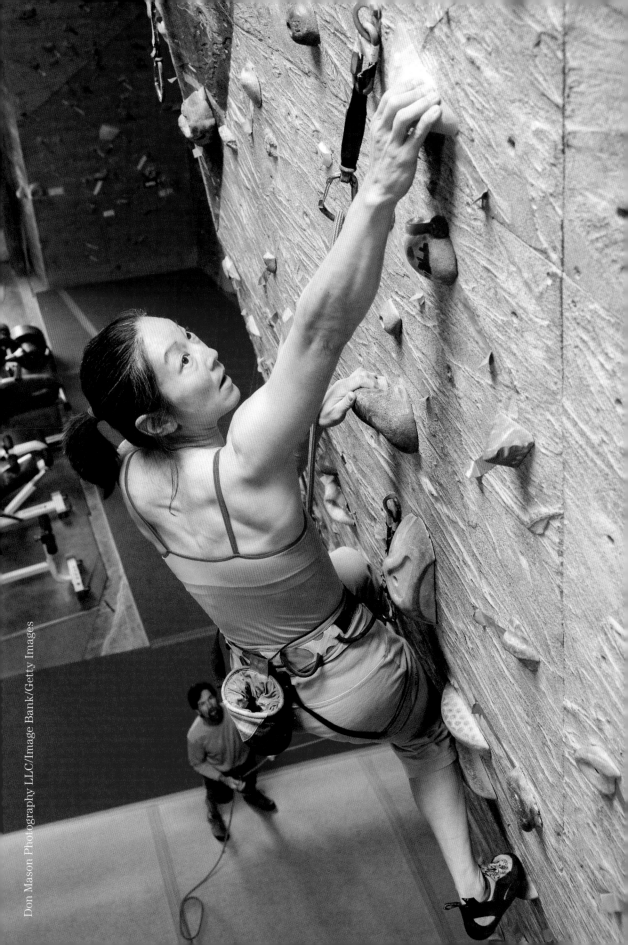

19

Goal Setting

Have you ever set a New Year's resolution that you didn't reach? Most likely you have—most of us have. Basically, what we tend to do is make one giant, nebulous goal ("I'm going to lose 30 pounds by the time my sister gets married!"). The problem is, we don't set up a roadmap to reach that goal, so we get lost on the way.

One of the most important habits you should implement when embarking on a health and fitness plan is to set goals. Proper goal setting has been shown to be a major key to success in most life endeavors, including fat loss. The cool thing about learning how to set good goals is that you can use these skills toward a lot of other things you may be trying to accomplish in your life, so bonus for you!

The basic goal-setting process looks kind of like this:

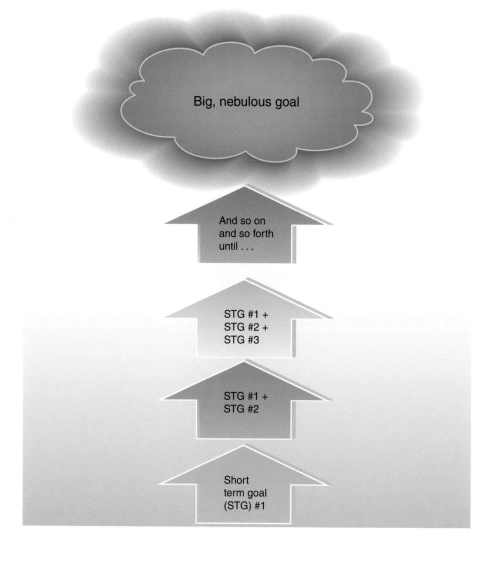

Your roadmap to your big, nebulous goal is made up of your short-term goals. Short-term goals are goals that can be reached within, say, one to three weeks. Your short-term goal should have the following qualifications:

- *Specific.* What, exactly, is your goal? How are you going to get it done? What will it require?

- *Measurable.* Can you quantify what you're doing? How will you measure it?

- *Attainable.* Is this a goal you're ready to take on right now? Do you have the skills and mental and emotional readiness to reach it?

- *Relevant.* Is this something that will help you get to your big, nebulous goal at the end? (If you're not sure, you might want to reevaluate what will help you.)

- *Time-bound.* Your goal should have a definite start date and end date.

These are called "SMART" goals, and I wish I had come up with this method myself, but I did not. The idea came from a guy named George Doran in a *Management Review* article in the early 1980s. Regardless, it's a very effective approach.

> *One of the most important habits you should implement when embarking on a health and fitness plan is to set goals.*

Let's use fat loss as an example, and let's say your big, nebulous goal is to lose 30 pounds. Ask yourself: What is one thing I am ready to do right now that will get me to that goal? Remember: It needs to be something you can manage within one to three weeks. It can be a mental health goal (maybe you need stress relief, for instance), a physical exercise goal, a physical health goal (maybe you don't sleep well, and that needs to be addressed), or a food goal.

So let's say you picked a food goal, and you picked, "I will eat more vegetables." Well, this is a little problematic. What's "more"? If you don't eat vegetables, and now you're eating some vegetables, then I guess that's more. But if you already eat vegetables, how do you know if you're eating more? Also, what kind of vegetables will you be eating more of? One kind? Lots of different kinds? This is what I mean by measurable. A better goal would be, "I will eat one serving of dark green leafy vegetables with every meal." Then you can say for sure you have or have not done this. If you went one meal without a dark-green leafy vegetable, then you did not reach this goal.

So, let's say you made your timeline three weeks, and you ate your green veggies with every meal for the whole time. If you feel good about this, and you are now comfortable with it, you're going to add a new goal. Keep the first goal—don't stop those habits. Your goals will be additive. So now you will have a serving of leafies with every meal, *and* you will, say, walk for one mile every day.

> *Reminding yourself of your goal on a regular basis can help you stick to it better.*

Suppose you don't reach your goal. In that case, keep that goal for the next round until you're comfortable with it. If you go two or three rounds without having reached this goal, you were not ready for it. Drop it for now and pick something that makes more sense for you at the moment.

When you set a goal, I think it helps to write it down, maybe in multiple places, preferably where you can see them often: put a Post-it on the fridge; write it on a notepad on your desk at work; tape a note to your bathroom mirror—whatever works. Reminding yourself of your goal on a regular basis can help you stick to it better.

The number of short-term goals you need to set in total depends entirely on how you implement them, and how big your ultimate goal is. However, this is generally not a fast process. I know that is frustrating. We all want everything *now*. But please understand that doing this in a manageable way will give you the best chance of getting long-term results, as opposed to jumping on a lose-weight-fast program and then gaining it all back again because you could not sustain that lifestyle.

Some people may be able to do two or three short-term goals at a time, and if you are one of those people, then go for it. However, I recommend one at a time for most people, as it is the easiest portion to manage. Fat loss can be a stressful process; don't make it harder on yourself than it needs to be.

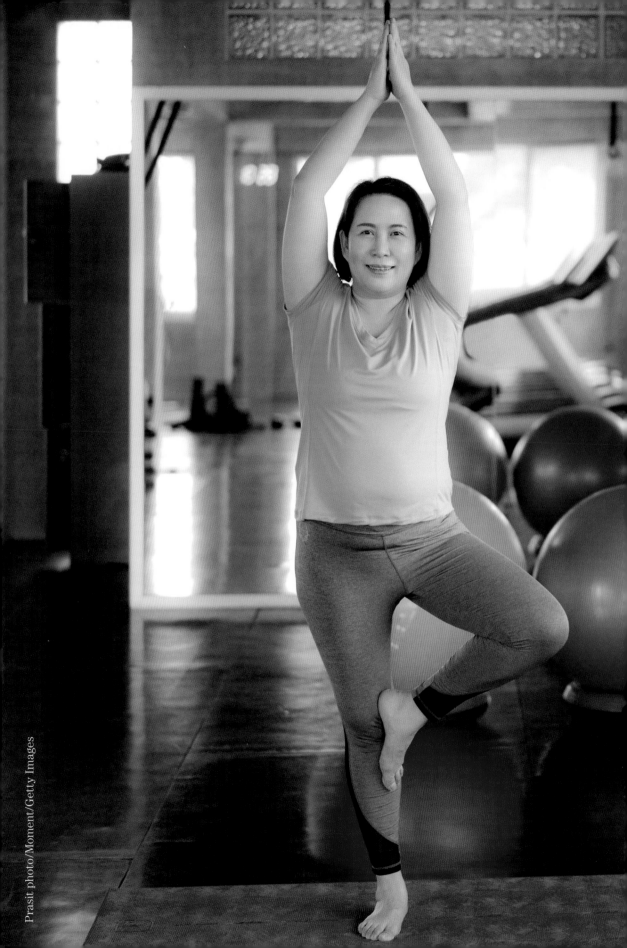

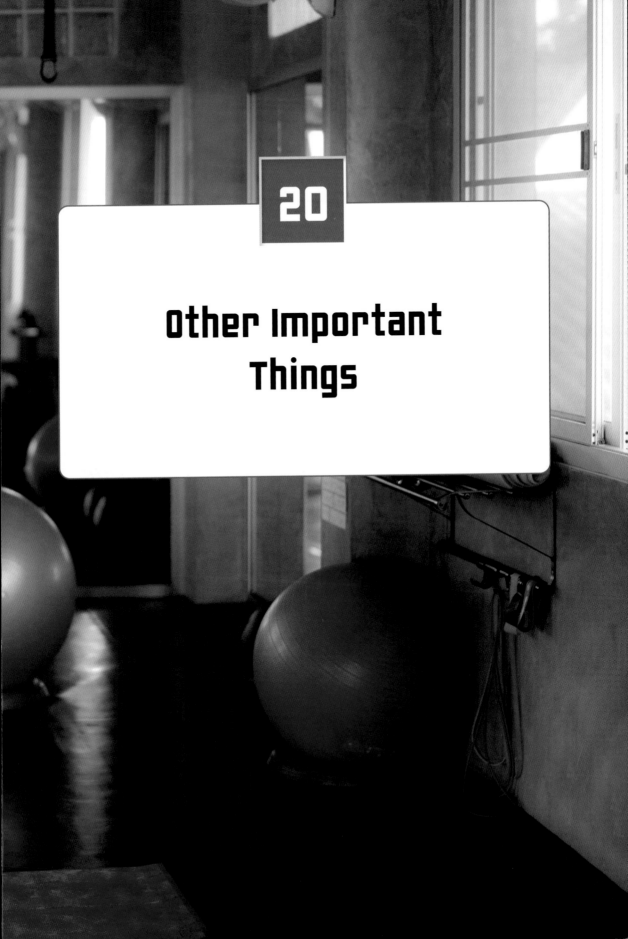

20

Other Important Things

There are several other factors that may impede fat loss that don't get talked about as much as they should. So let's talk about them!

SLEEP

I briefly touched on the importance of sleep earlier, but let's go a little deeper. When your body doesn't sleep well, a number of problems can occur. First, your brain doesn't function as it should (did you know, for instance, that driving while sleepy can be as dangerous as driving while drunk?). Also, your reflexes slow down, you don't perform well on mental or physical tasks, you get irritable, and everything pretty much sucks. Beyond that, your body does its best repairing while you're asleep. So if you're not sleeping well, your body won't repair well, and you won't get optimal results from your training program or from anything else.

When you don't sleep well, the hormones controlling your appetite go a little haywire, which can make you eat more. And, of course, excess calories lead to weight gain. Not sleeping much also leads to more hours awake, which leads to more eating opportunities, which leads to more calories, as well.

Speaking as someone who is in the bad-sleep club, I totally get how hard it is to figure out the secret to a good night's sleep. But I really recommend chasing after the answer to that secret. Great sleep is incredibly important to your overall mental, emotional, and physical health, as well as your fat loss goals.

STRESS

People who have high levels of chronic stress (caused by things like socioeconomic status, poor social networks, etc.) tend to be at a higher risk of obesity than those who do not have these stressors (206). This may be due to lowered exercise energy, comfort eating, access to more palatable foods (foods that are easy to eat a lot of, say, junk foods), and so on. Stress seems to affect the choices we make regarding the types of foods we eat and how much of them we eat. It is extremely important to find ways to mitigate stress levels and learn effective coping mechanisms to deal with life's stressors healthfully. A few methods that work for some include the following.

Meditation

Now, I'm not a big meditator; I've tried a million times and I just can't get my mind to shut up. I even took a meditation course at a Buddhist temple. But all I could think the whole time was that I had an itch, or that the floor was uncomfortable, or that I needed to switch my legs, and so on—not very zen. That being said, a lot of people swear by it, and there are many ways to meditate. What I found works best for me is walking in nature or by the ocean. It's not your typical *om*-type meditation, but it's a way for me to clear my head, appreciate something beautiful, and renew my perspective. Sometimes I take short walks, and sometimes I take much longer ones. I almost always bring my dog, as she loves it and is also a big sense of comfort to me. My point is that meditation doesn't have to take a traditional form if that doesn't work for you. Find a place of mental peace, whatever that is for you, and take the time to exercise that peace as often as possible.

Breathing Exercises

Deep-breathing exercises can be extremely useful as stress relievers. As a bonus, they can also help you learn how to breathe correctly for things like lifting and singing, so, hey, extra credit! There are various deep-breathing courses all over the Internet and potentially in your neighborhood. However, a simple one is this:

- Find a quiet, comfortable place and position. You can lie down or sit, whichever feels better.
- Place one hand on your chest and the other on your lower belly.
- Concentrate on filling your lower belly with air as you breathe in through your nose. Your shoulders shouldn't rise, and your upper hand should not expand very much—your lower hand should be doing most of the moving.
- Breathe out slowly and feel your lower belly start to relax again.
- Do this as many times as you feel you need for the time being.

If you like, you can try doing visualizations with your breathing exercises. Imagine yourself in your favorite, most relaxing place (Tahiti, anyone?), or think about your negative energy exiting your body every time you breathe out.

Exercise

Exercise has been shown to help mitigate anxiety, depression, and stress. However, the exercise's intensity matters. Moderate-intensity exercising appears to be the most effective at reducing inflammatory markers of stress (207), although most types of exercise seem to have at least some effect on depression markers and anxiety markers. Get out there and do something physical on a regular basis—it can make a huge difference.

Talk to Someone Supportive

Whether it's a qualified therapist, a spouse, a family member, or a trusted friend, talking about stress with a great, supportive listener can help improve coping mechanisms and can even improve the closeness in the relationship between you and the listener (if that's appropriate in your particular situation). Having a great support network doesn't come in handy only for fat loss; it helps with just about every area of life.

FINAL TRUTHS

Finally, I'd like to touch on a few things that seem to affect the way people view their own bodies. I'd be lying if these hadn't been things that have weighed on me in the past, as well. Hopefully, understanding these few things will help you cut yourself a little slack.

• *Just about everyone's stomach pooches out when they sit down.* I don't care if you're a supermodel—sitting down is not going to make your stomach look its best. I used to give myself a lot of grief over the way my stomach looked when I sat down. I'd grab on to whatever rolls formed and stress about them. But there are very, very few people whose stomachs don't form those godforsaken rolls when they sit down. So stop beating yourself up over that.

• *Lighting does amazing things.* If you're obsessing over the body of the Instagram influencer of your dreams, understand that lighting is everything in those pictures. The right lighting creates contours, highlights muscles, minimizes bulges, makes skin glow, and so on. A lot of people have become lighting experts with social media's advent, and these tricks have been used for ages by photographers to make their models look their best. This is also part of why you probably aren't thrilled with your bathing suit body in the store's dressing room. Those lights, in general, aren't exactly designed to flatter. It's kind of dumb on their part, if you think about it—they'd sell a lot more suits if they took a page out of the Good Lighting Handbook.

- *Even people with six-pack abs don't look like that all the time.* I remember I was talking to a popular fitness person a while back, and she was known for her amazing abs. "They don't always look like that, though," she lamented. "I really have to watch what I eat if I want my abs to pop." So while those people certainly have the genes, diet, body fat, and exercise plan that gives them their abs, everything still has to be perfect in order for them to look the way they do in pictures.

- Furthermore, *not everyone can have a six-pack (nor should everyone).* Having six-pack abs means having extremely low-enough body fat to see the musculature of the abdominal region, and that can be detrimental to one's health (i.e., can lead to amenorrhea, nutritional deficits, etc.). Of course, that doesn't happen to everyone, but it's certainly more common when one's body fat gets that low. There is also a genetic component to the six-pack abs. Personally, I don't have them. No matter how low I've gotten my body fat, the closest I've come to a six-pack was about a one-pack, and I looked emaciated.

> *Above all, your health, happiness, and mental well-being should be of the utmost priority.*

- *You will never have anyone else's body but yours.* So please, please stop comparing yourself to people in magazines, on social media, or anywhere else in the world. All you can do is make yourself the best "you" you can be. And you are the only one who can determine what that means for yourself. Above all, your health, happiness, and mental well-being should be of the utmost priority. I promise you, numbers on a scale or a flat stomach aren't necessarily the key to any of those things.

While losing fat can certainly be an important step toward good health and better self-image, there are many, many other factors that play into that, as well. So be good to yourself. Surround yourself with good people who want to help you be your best. Don't be afraid to seek out help when you need it, be it mental, physical, emotional, or otherwise. Understand that you are not alone in your quest for self-improvement, and there will always be others in your corner.

POSTSCRIPT

This book was basically a massive brain-dump of information with the purpose of answering as factually as possible the questions relating to fat loss I see and hear every day. The cool thing about the study of nutrition and food psychology is that the landscape is always changing—there's always new information to learn about. Unfortunately, with the advent of the Internet and social media, we have a glut of great information and not-so-great information, and it isn't always easy to understand it all. Certain people have much to gain by selling a specific product or dogma, and the sad side effect is that many people are swindled out of their money (and potentially their health) as a result. In this book, I hoped to clear up some of that mess and give you as many tools as possible to help you navigate through the muck. I hope you have found it useful and that you continue to be a steward of your own health, as difficult and uncomfortable as that can be sometimes.

I look forward to your success.

REFERENCES

1. Astrup, A., Larsen, T.M., & Harper, A. (2004). Atkins and other low-carbohydrate diets: hoax or an effective tool for weight loss? *The Lancet, 364*(9437), 897-899. doi:10.1016/s0140-6736(04)16986-9

2. Johnston, B.C., Kanters, S., Bandayrel, K., Wu, P., Naji, F., Siemieniuk, R.A., . . . Mills, E.J. (2014). Comparison of weight loss among named diet programs in overweight and obese adults. *JAMA, 312*(9), 923. doi:10.1001/jama.2014.10397

3. Naude, C.E., Schoonees, A., Senekal, M., Young, T., Garner, P., & Volmink, J. (2014). Low carbohydrate versus isoenergetic balanced diets for reducing weight and cardiovascular risk: a systematic review and meta-analysis. *PLoS ONE, 9*(7). doi:10.1371/journal.pone.0100652

4. Soenen, S., & Westerterp-Plantenga, M.S. (2008). Proteins and satiety: implications for weight management. *Current Opinion in Clinical Nutrition and Metabolic Care, 11*(6), 747-751. doi:10.1097/mco.0b013e328311a8c4

5. Gibson, A.A., Seimon, R.V., Lee, C.M., Ayre, J., Franklin, J., Markovic, T.P., . . . Sainsbury, A. (2014). Do ketogenic diets really suppress appetite? A systematic review and meta-analysis. *Obesity Reviews, 16*(1), 64-76. doi:10.1111/obr.12230

6. Dhillon, J., Craig, B.A., Leidy, H.J., Amankwaah, A.F., Anguah, K.O., Jacobs, A., . . . Tucker, R.M. (2016). The effects of increased protein intake on fullness: a meta-analysis and its limitations. *Journal of the Academy of Nutrition and Dietetics, 116*(6), 968-983. doi:10.1016/j.jand.2016.01.003

7. Anton, S., Hida, A., Heekin, K., Sowalsky, K., Karabetian, C., Mutchie, H., . . . Barnett, T. (2017). Effects of popular diets without specific calorie targets on weight loss outcomes: systematic review of findings from clinical trials. *Nutrients, 9*(8), 822. doi:10.3390/nu9080822

8. Jenkins, D.J., Wong, J.M., Kendall, C.W., Esfahani, A., Ng, V.W., Leong, T.C., . . . Singer, W. (2014). Effect of a 6-month vegan low-carbohydrate ("Eco-Atkins") diet on cardiovascular risk factors and body weight in hyperlipidaemic adults: a randomised controlled trial. *BMJ Open, 4*(2). doi:10.1136/bmjopen-2013-003505

9. Neacsu, M., Fyfe, C., Horgan, G., & Johnstone, A.M. (2014). Appetite control and biomarkers of satiety with vegetarian (soy) and meat-based high-protein diets for weight loss in obese men: a randomized crossover trial. *American Journal of Clinical Nutrition, 100*(2), 548-558. doi:10.3945/ajcn.113.077503

10. Hall, K., Bemis, T., Brychta, R., Chen, K., Courville, A., Crayner, E., . . . Yannai, L. (2015). Calorie for calorie, dietary fat restriction results in more body fat loss than carbohydrate restriction in people with obesity. *Cell Metabolism, 22*(3), 531. doi:10.1016/j.cmet.2015.08.009

11. Sutton, E.F., Bray, G.A., Burton, J.H., Smith, S.R., & Redman, L.M. (2016). No evidence for metabolic adaptation in thermic effect of food by dietary protein. *Obesity, 24*(8), 1639-1642. doi:10.1002/oby.21541

12. Antonio, J., Peacock, C.A., Ellerbroek, A., Fromhoff, B., & Silver, T. (2014). The effects of consuming a high protein diet (4.4 g/kg/d) on body composition in resistance-trained individuals. *Journal of the International Society of Sports Nutrition, 11*(1), 19. doi:10.1186/1550-2783-11-19

13. Li, J., Armstrong, C., & Campbell, W. (2016). Effects of dietary protein source and quantity during weight loss on appetite, energy expenditure, and cardio-metabolic responses. *Nutrients, 8*(2), 63. doi:10.3390/nu8020063

14. Leidy, H.J., Clifton, P.M., Astrup, A., Wycherley, T.P., Westerterp-Plantenga, M.S., Luscombe-Marsh, N.D. . . . & Mattes, S. (2015). The role of protein in weight loss and maintenance. *The American Journal of Clinical Nutrition, 101*(6), 1320S-1329S. doi:10.3945/ajcn.114.084038

15. Atallah, R., Filion, K.B., Wakil, S.M., Genest, J., Joseph, L., Poirier, P., . . . Eisenberg, M.J. (2014). Long-term effects of 4 popular diets on weight loss and cardiovascular risk factors: A systematic review of randomized controlled trials. *Circulation: Cardiovascular Quality and Outcomes, 7*(6), 815-827. doi:10.1161/circoutcomes.113.000723

16. Kosinski, C., & Jornayvaz, F. (2017). Effects of ketogenic diets on cardiovascular risk factors: evidence from animal and human studies. *Nutrients, 9*(6), 517. doi:10.3390/nu9050517

17. Eyres, L., Eyres, M.F., Chisholm, A., & Brown, R.C. (2016). Coconut oil consumption and cardiovascular risk factors in humans. *Nutrition Reviews, 74*(4), 267-280. doi:10.1093/nutrit/nuw002

18. Hruby, A., & Hu, F.B. (2016). Saturated fat and heart disease: The latest evidence. *Lipid Technology, 28*(1), 7-12. doi:10.1002/lite.201600001

19. Nettleton, J.A., Brouwer, I.A., Geleijnse, J.M., & Hornstra, G. (2017). Saturated fat consumption and risk of coronary heart disease and ischemic stroke: A science update. *Annals of Nutrition and Metabolism, 70*(1), 26-33. doi:10.1159/000455681

20. Wang, X., Lin, X., Ouyang, Y.Y., Liu, J., Zhao, G., Pan, A., & Hu, F.B. (2015). Red and processed meat consumption and mortality: dose–response meta-analysis of prospective cohort studies. *Public Health Nutrition, 19*(05), 893-905. doi:10.1017/s1368980015002062

21. Domingo, J.L., & Nadal, M. (2017). Carcinogenicity of consumption of red meat and processed meat: A review of scientific news since the IARC decision. *Food and Chemical Toxicology, 105*, 256-261. doi:10.1016/j.fct.2017.04.028

22. Clegg, M.E. (2017). They say coconut oil can aid weight loss, but can it really? *European Journal of Clinical Nutrition, 71*(10), 1139-1143. doi:10.1038/ejcn.2017.86

23. Mumme, K., & Stonehouse, W. (2015). Effects of medium-chain triglycerides on weight loss and body composition: A meta-analysis of randomized controlled trials. *Journal of the Academy of Nutrition and Dietetics, 115*(2), 249-263. doi:10.1016/j.jand.2014.10.022

24. Bueno, N.B., Melo, I.V., Florêncio, T.T., & Sawaya, A.L. (2015). Dietary medium-chain triacylglycerols versus long-chain triacylglycerols for body composition in adults: Systematic review and meta-analysis of randomized controlled trials. *Journal of the American College of Nutrition, 34*(2), 175-183. doi:10.1080/07315724.2013.879844

25. Dinicolantonio, J.J. (2014). The cardiometabolic consequences of replacing saturated fats with carbohydrates or \gV\-6 polyunsaturated fats: Do the dietary guidelines have it wrong? *Open Heart, 1*(1). doi:10.1136/openhrt-2013-000032

26. Souza, R.J., Mente, A., Maroleanu, A., Cozma, A.I., Ha, V., Kishibe, T., . . . Anand, S.S. (2015). Intake of saturated and trans unsaturated fatty acids and risk of all cause mortality, cardiovascular disease, and type 2 diabetes: Systematic review and meta-analysis of observational studies. *Bmj, 351*. doi:10.1136/bmj.h3978

27. Wang, D.D., Li, Y., Chiuve, S.E., Stampfer, M.J., Manson, J.E., Rimm, E.B., . . . Hu, F.B. (2016). Association of specific dietary fats with total and cause-specific mortality. *JAMA Internal Medicine, 176*(8), 1134. doi:10.1001/jamainternmed.2016.2417

28. Jakobsen, M.U., Dethlefsen, C., Joensen, A.M., Stegger, J., Tjønneland, A., Schmidt, E.B., & Overvad, K. (2010). Intake of carbohydrates compared with intake of saturated fatty acids and risk of myocardial infarction; importance of the glycemic index. *American Journal of Clinical Nutrition, 91*(6), 1764-1768. doi:10.3945/ajcn.2009.29099

29. Briggs, M., Petersen, K., & Kris-Etherton, P. (2017). Saturated fatty acids and cardiovascular disease: replacements for saturated fat to reduce cardiovascular risk. *Healthcare, 5*(2), 29. doi:10.3390/healthcare5020029

30. Kris-Etherton, P.M., & Fleming, J.A. (2015). Emerging Nutrition Science on Fatty Acids and Cardiovascular Disease: Nutritionists Perspectives. *Advances in Nutrition: An International Review Journal, 6*(3). doi:10.3945/an.114.006981

31. Berge, A.F. (2007). How the ideology of low fat conquered America. *Journal of the History of Medicine and Allied Sciences, 63*(2), 139-177. doi:10.1093/jhmas/jrn001

32. Condor, B. (1997, May 8). "Heart-Healthy" label is for sale. *Chicago Tribune.* Retrieved from http://articles.orlandosentinel.com/1997-05-08/lifestyle/9705060420_1_heart-frosted-flakes-fat

33. National Institute of Diabetes and Digestive and Kidney Diseases. *Overweight and Obesity Statistics.* Retrieved from www.niddk.nih.gov/health-information/health-statistics/overweight-obesity

34. Ford, E.S., Ajani, M.B., Croft, J.B., Critchley, J.A., Labarthe, D.R., Kottke, T.E., . . . & Capewell, S. (2007). Explaining the decrease in US deaths from coronary disease, 1980-2000. *Survey of Anesthesiology, 51*(6), 326. doi:10.1097/sa.0b013e31815c1098

35. Hall, K.D., & Guo, J. (2017). Obesity energetics: body weight regulation and the effects of diet composition. *Gastroenterology, 152*(7). doi:10.1053/j.gastro.2017.01.052

36. Nordmann, A.J., Nordmann, A., Briel, M., Keller, U., Yancy, W.S. & Bucher, H.C. (2006). Effects of low-carbohydrate vs. low-fat diets on weight loss and cardiovascular risk factors: A meta-analysis of randomized controlled trials. *Archives of Internal Medicine* (166).

37. Tobias, D.K., Chen, M., Manson, J.E., Ludwig, D.S., Willett, W., & Hu, F.B. (2015). Effect of low-fat diet interventions versus other diet interventions on long-term weight change in adults: a systematic review and meta-analysis. *The Lancet Diabetes & Endocrinology, 3*(12), 968-979. doi:10.1016/s2213-8587(15)00367-8

38. Siri-Tarino, P.W., Chiu, S., Bergeron, N., & Krauss, R.M. (2015). Saturated fats versus polyunsaturated fats versus carbohydrates for cardiovascular disease prevention and treatment. *Annual Review of Nutrition, 35*(1), 517-543. doi:10.1146/annurev-nutr-071714-034449

39. Dinicolantonio, J.J., Lucan, S.C., & O'Keefe, J.H. (2016). The evidence for saturated fat and for sugar related to coronary heart disease. *Progress in Cardiovascular Diseases, 58*(5), 464-472. doi:10.1016/j.pcad.2015.11.006

40. Oregon State University, Linus Pauling Institute Micronutrient Information Center. *Essential Fatty Acids.* Retrieved from http://lpi.oregonstate.edu/mic/other-nutrients/essential-fatty-acids

41. Mogensen, K.M. (2017). *Essential Fatty Acid Deficiency.* Retrieved from https://med.virginia.edu/ginutrition/wp-content/uploads/sites/199/2014/06/Parrish-June-17.pdf

42. Seal, C.J., & Brownlee, I.A. (2015). Whole-grain foods and chronic disease: Evidence from epidemiological and intervention studies. *Proceedings of the Nutrition Society, 74*(03), 313-319. doi:10.1017/s0029665115002104

43. Kiens, B., & Astrup, A. (2015). Ketogenic diets for fat loss and exercise performance. *Exercise and Sport Sciences Reviews, 43*(3), 109. doi:10.1249/jes.0000000000000053

44. Paoli, A., Bianco, A., & Grimaldi, K.A. (2015). The ketogenic diet and sport: A possible marriage? *Exercise and Sport Sciences Reviews, 43*(3), 153-162. doi:10.1249/jes.0000000000000050

45. Mcevedy, S.M., Sullivan-Mort, G., Mclean, S.A., Pascoe, M.C., & Paxton, S.J. (2017). Ineffectiveness of commercial weight-loss programs for achieving modest but meaningful weight loss: Systematic review and meta-analysis. *Journal of Health Psychology, 22*(12), 1614-1627. doi:10.1177/1359105317705983

46. Finkelstein, E.A., & Kruger, E. (2014). Meta- and cost-effectiveness analysis of commercial weight loss strategies. *Obesity, 22*(9), 1942-1951. doi:10.1002/oby.20824

47. Gudzune, K.A., Doshi, R.S., Mehta, A.K., Chaudhry, Z.W., Jacobs, D.K., Vakil, R.M., . . . Clark, J.M. (2015). Efficacy of Commercial Weight-Loss Programs. *Annals of Internal Medicine, 162*(7), 501. doi:10.7326/m14-2238

48. Fenton, K.L. (2017). Unpacking the sustainability of meal kit delivery: A comparative analysis of energy use, carbon emissions, and related costs for meal kit services and grocery stores. *University of Texas at Austin Texas ScholarWorks*. Retrieved from https://repositories.lib.utexas.edu/handle/2152/61651

49. Bennett, W.L., & Appel, L.J. (2015). Vegetarian diets for weight loss: How strong is the evidence? *Journal of General Internal Medicine, 31*(1), 9-10. doi:10.1007/s11606-015-3471-7

50. Turner-McGrievy, G., Mandes, T., & Crimarco, A. (2017). A plant-based diet for overweight and obesity prevention and treatment. *Journal of Geriatric Cardiology, 14*(5), 369-374. doi:10.11909/j.issn.1671-5411.2017.05.002

51. Gibson, A.A., Seimon, R.V., Lee, C.M., Ayre, J., Franklin, J., Markovic, T.P., & Sainsbury, A. (2014). Do ketogenic diets really suppress appetite? A systematic review and meta-analysis. *Obesity Reviews, 16*(1), 64-76. doi:10.1111/obr.12230

52. Emadian, A., Andrews, R.C., England, C.Y., Wallace, V., & Thompson, J.L. (2015). The effect of macronutrients on glycaemic control: A systematic review of dietary randomised controlled trials in overweight and obese adults with type 2 diabetes in which there was no difference in weight loss between treatment groups. *British Journal of Nutrition, 114*(10), 1656-1666. doi:10.1017/s0007114515003475

53. Brownlee, I.A., Chater, P.I., Pearson, J.P., & Wilcox, M.D. (2017). Dietary fibre and weight loss: Where are we now? *Food Hydrocolloids, 68*, 186-191. doi:10.1016/j.foodhyd.2016.08.029

54. Huang, R.Y., Huang, C.C., Hu, F.B., & Chavarro, J.E. (2016). Vegetarian diets and weight reduction: A meta-analysis of randomized controlled trials. *Journal of General Internal Medicine, 31*(1), 109-166.

55. Cook, A. (2000). The problem of accuracy in dietary surveys. Analysis of the over 65 UK National Diet and Nutrition Survey. *Journal of Epidemiology & Community Health, 54*(8), 611-616. doi:10.1136/jech.54.8.611

56. Archer, E., Hand, G.A., & Blair, S.N. (2013). Validity of U.S. nutritional surveillance: National health and nutrition examination survey caloric energy intake data, 1971-2010. *PLOS ONE, 8*(10). doi:10.1371/journal.pone.0076632

57. Dinu, M., Abbate, R., Gensini, G.F., Casini, A., & Sofi, F. (2016). Vegetarian, vegan diets and multiple health outcomes: A systematic review with meta-analysis of observational studies. *Critical Reviews in Food Science and Nutrition, 57*(17), 3640-3649. doi:10.1080/10408398.2016.1138447

58. Kim, H., Caulfield, L.E., & Rebholz, C.M. (2018). Healthy plant-based diets are associated with lower risk of all-cause mortality in US adults. *The Journal of Nutrition, 148*(4), 624-631. doi:10.1093/jn/nxy019

59. Song, M., Fung, T.T., Hu, F.B., Willett, W.C., Longo, V.D., Chan, A.T., & Giovannucci, E.L. (2016). Association of animal and plant protein intake with all-cause and cause-specific mortality. *JAMA Internal Medicine, 176*(10), 1453. doi:10.1001/jamainternmed.2016.4182

60. Craddock, J.C., Probst, Y.C., & Peoples, G.E. (2016). Vegetarian and omnivorous nutrition—Comparing physical performance. *Human Kinetics Journals, 26*(3), 212-220. doi:10.1123/ijsnem.2015-0231

61. Lopez, P.D., Cativo, E.H., Atlas, S.A., & Rosendorff, C. (2019). The effect of vegan diets on blood pressure in adults: A meta-analysis of randomized controlled trials. *The American Journal of Medicine, 132*(7), 875-883.e7.

62. Melina, V., Craig, W., & Levin, S. (2016). Position of the Academy of Nutrition and Dietetics: Vegetarian diets. *Journal of the Academy of Nutrition and Dietetics, 116*(12), 1970-1980.

63. Richter, M., Boeing, H., Grünewald-Funk, D., Heseker, H., Kroke, A., Leschik-Bonnet, E., . . . Watzl, B. (2016). Vegan diets. *Ernahrungs Umschau* 63(4): 92-102. Erratum in: *63*(5): M262.

64. Agnoli, C., Baroni, L., Bertini, I., Ciappellano, S., Fabbri, A., Papa, M., . . . Sieri, S. (2017). Position paper on vegetarian diets of the Italian Society of Human Nutrition. *Nutrition, Metabolism, and Cardiovascular Diseases, 27*(12), 1037-1052. doi:10.1016/j.numecd.2017.10.020

65. Tan, C., Zhao, Y., & Wang, S. (2018). Is a vegetarian diet safe to follow during pregnancy? A systematic review and meta-analysis of observational studies. *Critical Reviews in Food Science and Nutrition.* doi:10.1080/10408398.2018.1461062

66. Piccoli, G.B., Clari, R., Vigotti, F.N., Leone, F., Attini, R., Cabiddu, G., . . . Avagnina, P. (2015). Vegan-vegetarian diets in pregnancy: danger or panacea? A systematic narrative review. *BJOG, 122*(5), 623-633. doi:10.1111/1471-0528.13280

67. Nieman, D.C. (1999). Physical fitness and vegetarian diets: Is there a relation? *American Journal of Clinical Nutrition, 70*(3 Suppl), 570S-575S. doi:10.1093/ajcn/70.3.570s.

68. Hanne, N., Dlin, R., & Rotstein, A. (1986). Physical fitness, anthropometric and metabolic parameters in vegetarian athletes. *Journal of Sports Medicine and Physical Fitness, 26*(2), 180-185.

69. Campbell, W.W., Barton, M.L., Cyr-Campbell, D., Davey, S.L., Beard, J.L., Parise, G., & Evans, W.J. (1999). Effects of an omnivorous diet compared with a lactoovovegetarian diet on resistance-training-induced changes in body composition and skeletal muscle in older men. *American Journal of Clinical Nutrition. 70*(6), 1032-1039.

70. Haub, M.D., Wells, A.M., Tarnopolsky, M.A., & Campbell, W.W. (2002). Effect of protein source on resistive-training-induced changes in body composition and muscle size in older men. *American Journal of Clinical Nutrition, 76*(3), 511-517.

71. Koebnick, C., Strassner, C., Hoffmann, I., & Leitzmann, C. (1999). Consequences of a long-term raw food diet on body weight and menstruation: Results of a questionnaire study. *Annals of Nutrition & Metabolism, 43*, 69-79.

72. Groopman, E.E., Carmody, R.N., & Wrangham, R.W. (2015). Cooking increases net energy gain from a lipid-rich food. *American Journal of Physical Anthropology. 156*(1), 11-18.

73. Carmody, R.N., Weintraub, G.S., & Wrangham, R.W. (2011). Energetic consequences of thermal and nonthermal food processing. *Proceedings of the National Academy of Sciences of the United States of America, 108*(48), 19199-19203. doi:10.1073/pnas.1112128108

74. Garcia, A.L., Koebnick, C., Dagnelie, P.C., Strassner, C., Elmadfa, I., Katz, N., . . . Hoffman, I. (2008). Long-term strict raw food diet is associated with favourable plasma and low plasma lycopene in Germans. *British Journal of Nutrition, 99*(6), 1293-1300.

75. Cunningham, E. (2004). What is a raw foods diet and are there any risks or benefits associated with it? *Journal of the Academy of Nutrition and Dietetics, 104*(10), 1623.

76. Miglio, C., Chiavaro, E., Visconti, A., Fogliano, V., & Pellegrini, N. (2008). Effects of different cooking methods on nutritional and physicochemical characteristics of selected vegetables. *Journal of Agriculture and Food Chemistry, 56*(1), 139-147.

77. Fabbri, A.D.T., Crosby, G.A. (2016). A review of the impact of preparation and cooking on the nutritional quality of vegetables and legumes. *International Journal of Gastronomy and Food Science, 3*, 2-11.

78. Fontana, L., Shew, J.L., & Holloszy, J.O. (2005). Low bone mass in subjects on a long-term raw vegetarian diet. *JAMA Internal Medicine, 165*(6), 684-689. doi:10.1001/archinte.165.6.684

79. Minihane, A.M., Vinoy, S., Russell, W.R., Baka, A., Roche, H.M., Tuohy, K.M., . . . Calder, P. (2015). Low-grade inflammation, diet composition, and health: Current research evidence and its translation. *British Journal of Nutrition, 114*, 999-1012. doi:10.1017/S0007114515002093

80. Misiak, B., Leszek, J., & Kiejna, A. (2012). Metabolic syndrome, mild cognitive impairment and Alzheimer's disease—The emerging role of systemic low-grade inflammation and adiposity. *Brain Research Bulletin, 89*(3-4), 144-149.

81. Ruiz-Nuñez, B., Pruimboom, L., Janneke Dijck-Brouwer, D.A., & Muskiet, F.A.J. (2013). Lifestyle and nutritional imbalances associated with Western diseases: Causes and consequences of chronic systemic low-grade inflammation in an evolutionary context. *The Journal of Nutritional Biochemistry, 24*(7), 1183-1201.

82. Harris, L., Hamilton, S., Azevedo, L.B., Olajide, J., De Brún, C., Waller, G., . . . Ells, L. (2018). Intermittent fasting interventions for treatment of overweight and obesity in adults: A systematic review and meta-analysis. *JBI Database of Systematic Reviews and Implementation Reports, 16*(2), 507-547. doi:10.11124/JBISRIR-2016-003248

83. Varady, K.A. (2011). Intermittent vs. daily caloric restriction: Which diet regimen is more effective for weight loss? *Obesity Reviews, 12*(7), E593-E601. doi:10.1111/j.1467-789X.2011.00873.x

84. Anton, S.D., Moehl, K., Donahoo, W.T., Marosi, K., Lee, S.A., Mainous, A.G., Leeuwenburgh, C., & Mattson, M.P. (2017). Flipping the metabolic switch: Understanding and applying the health benefits of fasting. *Obesity, 26*(2), 254-268. doi:10.1002/oby.22065

85. Golbidi, S., Daiber, A., Korac, B., Li, H., Essop, M.F., & Laher, I. (2017). Health benefits of fasting and caloric restriction. *Current Diabetes Reports, 17*(123), doi:10.1007/s11892-017-0951-7

86. Levy, E., & Chu, T. (2019). Intermittent fasting and its effects on athletic performance: A review. *Current Sports Medicine Reports, 18*(7), 266-269. doi:10.1249/JSR.0000000000000614

87. Statista. Gluten-free and free-from food retail sales in the United States from 2006 to 2020 (in billion U.S. dollars). Retrieved November 21, 2019, from www.statista.com/statistics/261099/us-gluten-free-and-free-from-retail-sales

88. Topper, A. Non-celiacs Drive Gluten-Free Market Growth. Mintel Group Ltd. Web. Retrieved November 21, 2019, from www.mintel.com/blog/food-market-news/gluten-free-consumption-trends

89. Kim, H-S, Demyen, M.S., Mathew, J., Kothari, N., Feurdean, M., & Ahlawat, S.K. (2017). Obesity, metabolic syndrome and cardiovascular risk in gluten-free followers without celiac disease in the United States: results from the National Health and Nutrition Examination Survey 2009–2014. *Digestive Diseases and Sciences, 62*(9), 2440-2448.

90. Niland, B., & Cash, B.D. (2018). Health benefits and adverse effects of a gluten-free diet in non-celiac disease patients. *Gastroenterology & Hepatology, 14*(2), 82-91.

91. Lebwohl, B., Cao, Y., Zong, G., Hu, F., Green, P.H.R., Neugut, A.I., . . . Chan, A.T. Long term gluten consumption in adults without celiac disease and risk of coronary heart disease: prospective cohort study. (2017). *BMJ, 357*(j1892). doi:10.1136/bmj.j1892

92. Liu, P.H., Lebwohl, B., Burke, K.E., Ivey, K.L., Ananthakrishnan, A.N., Lochhead, P., . . . Khalili, H. (2019) Dietary gluten intake and risk of microscopic colitis among US women without celiac disease: A prospective cohort study. *Gastroenterology, 114*(1), 127-134. doi:10.1038/s41395-018-0267-5

93. Zong, G., Lebwohl, B., Hu, F.B., Sampson, L., Doughtery, L.W., Willett, W.C., . . . Sun, Q. (2018). Gluten intake and risk of type 2 diabetes in three large prospective cohort studies of US men and women. *Diabetologia, 61*(10), 2164-2173.

94. Um, C.Y., Campbell, P.T., Carter, B., Wang, Y., Gapstur, S.M., & McCullough, M.L. (2019). Association between grains, gluten, and the risk of colorectal cancer in the cancer prevention study- II nutrition cohort. *European Journal of Nutrition,* epub ahead of print. doi:10.1007/s00394-019-02032-2

95. Vici, G., Belli, L., Biondi, M., & Polzonetti, V. (2016). Gluten free diet and nutrient deficiencies: A review. *Clinical Nutrition, 35*, 136-1241.

96. Cusack, L., De Buck, E., Compernolle, V., & Vandekerckhove, P. (2013). Blood type diets lack supporting evidence: A systematic review. *The American Journal of Clinical Nutrition, 98*(1), 99-104. doi:10.3945/ajcn.113.058693

97. Wang, J., García-Bailo, B., Nielsen, D.E., & El-Sohemy, A. (2014). *ABO* genotype, "Blood-Type" diet and cardiometabolic risk factors. *PLOS One.* doi:10.1371/journal.pone.0084749

98. Wang, J., Jamnik, J., García-Bailo, B., Nielsen, D.E, Kenkins, D.J.A., & El-Sohemy, A. (2018). ABO genotype does not modify the association between the "Blood-Type" diet and biomarkers of cardiometabolic disease in overweight adults. *The Journal of Nutrition, 148*(4), 518-525. doi:10.1093/jn/nxx074

99. Mackie, G.M., Samocha-Bonet, D., & Tam, C.S. (2017). Does weight cycling promote obesity and metabolic risk factors? *Obesity Research & Clinical Practice, 11*(2), 131-139. doi:10.1016/j.orcp.2016.10.284

100. Rothblum, E.D. (2018). Slim chance for permanent weight loss. *Archives of Scientific Psychology, 6*(1), 63-69. doi:10.1037/arc0000043

101. Klein, A.V., & Kiat, H. (2014). Detox diets for toxin elimination and weight management: A critical review of the evidence. *Journal of Human Nutrition and Dietetics.* doi:10.1111/jhn.12286

102. Mancini, J.G., Filion, K.B., Atallah, R., & Eisenberg, M.J. (2016). Systematic review of the Mediterranean diet for long-term weight loss. *The American Journal of Medicine, 129*(4), 407-415.e4. doi:10.1016/j.amjmed.2015.11.028

103. Esposito, K., Kastorini, C.M., Panagiotakos, D.B., & Giugliano, D. (2011). Mediterranean diet and weight loss: Meta-analysis of randomized controlled trials. *Metabolic Syndrome and Related Disorders, 9*(1), 1-12.

104. Huo, R., Du, T., Xu, W., Chen, X., Sun, K., & Yu, X. (2015). Effects of Mediterranean-style diet on glycemic control, weight loss, and cardiovascular risk factors among type 2 diabetes individuals: A meta-analysis. *European Journal of Clinical Nutrition, 69*(11), 1200-1208. doi:0.1038/ejcn.2014.243

105. Castro-Barquero, S., Lamuela-Raventós, R.M., Doménech, M., & Estruch, R. (2018). Relationship between Mediterranean dietary polyphenol intake and obesity. *Nutrients, 10*(10), 1523. doi:10.3390/nu10101523

106. Passos de Jesus, R., Mota, J.F., González-Muniesa, P., Linetzky Waitzberg, D., Marques Telles, M., & Amador Bueno, A. (2018). Plant polyphenols in obesity and obesity-related metabolic disorders: A narrative review of resveratrol and flavonoids upon the molecular basis of inflammation. *Journal of Obesity and Nutritional Disorders.* doi:10.29011/2577-2244.100029

107. Aragon, A.A., & Schoenfeld, B.J. (2013). Nutrient timing revisited: Is there a post-exercise anabolic window? *Journal of the International Society of Sports Nutrition, 10*(5). doi:10.1186/1550-2783-10-5

108. Schoenfeld, B.J., Aragon, A.A., & Krieger, J.W. (2015). Effects of meal frequency on weight loss and body composition: A meta-analysis. *Nutrition Reviews, 73*(2), 69-82. doi:10.1093/nutrit/nuu017

109. Perrigue, M.M., Drewnowski, A., Wang, C.Y., & Neuhouser, M.L. (2015). Higher eating frequency does not increase appetite in healthy adults. *The Journal of Nutrition, 146*(1), 59-64. doi:10.3945/jn.115.216978

110. Minerals in Himalayan pink salt: Spectral analysis. Retrieved December 26, 2019, from https://themeadow.com/pages/minerals-in-himalayan-pink-salt-spectral-analysis

111. Drake, S.L., & Drake, M.A. (2010). Comparison of salty taste and time intensity of sea and land salts from around the world. *Journal of Sensory Studies, 26*(1). doi:10.1111/j.1745-459X.2010.00317.x

112. National Institutes of Health Office of Dietary Supplements: Calcium Fact Sheet for Health Professionals. Retrieved December 26, 2019, from https://ods.od.nih.gov/factsheets/Calcium-HealthProfessional

113. National Institutes of Health Office of Dietary Supplements: Iodine Fact Sheet for Health Professionals. Retrieved December 26, 2019, from https://ods.od.nih.gov/factsheets/Iodine-HealthProfessional

114. Vigar, V., Myers, S., Oliver, C., Arellano, J., Robinson, S., & Leifert, C. (2019). A systematic review of organic versus conventional food consumption: Is there a measurable benefit on human health? *Nutrients, 12*(1), 7. doi:10.3390/nu12010007

115. Electronic Code of Federal Regulations. Retrieved December 27, 2019, from www.ecfr.gov/cgi-bin/text-idx?c=ecfr&SID=9874504b6f1025eb0e6b67cadf9d3b40&rgn=div6&view=text&node=7:3.1.1.9.32.7&idno=7

116. Formal Recommendation From: National Organic Standards Board (NOSB) To: The National Organic Program (NOP). Retrieved December 27, 2019, from www.ams.usda.gov/sites/default/files/media/Rotenone%20recommendation%202012.pdf

117. World Health Organization. WHO answers questions on genetically modified foods. Retrieved December 27, 2019, from www.who.int/mediacentre/news/notes/np5/en

118. National Academies of Sciences, Engineering, and Medicine. (2016). Report: Genetically engineered crops: Experiences and Prospects. Retrieved December 27, 2019, from http://nas-sites.org/ge-crops/category/report

119. Hilbeck, A., Binimelis, R., Defarge, N., Steinbrecher, R., Székács, A., Wickson, F., . . . Wynne, B. (2015). No scientific consensus on GMO safety. *Environmental Sciences Europe, 27*(4).

120. Wallace, T., Murray, R., & Zelman, K.M. (2016). The nutritional value and health benefits of chickpeas and hummus. *Nutrients, 8*(12), 766.

121. Rebello, C.J., Greenway, F.L., & Finley, J.W. (2014). A review of the nutritional value of legumes and their effects on obesity and its related co-morbidities. *Obesity Reviews, 15*(5), 392-407. doi:10.1111/obr.12144

122. Sharma, S.P., Chung, H.J., Kim, H.J., & Hong, S.T. (2016). Paradoxical effects of fruit on obesity. *Nutrients, 8*(10), 633. doi:10.3390/nu8100633

123. Smith, J., & Wang, F. (2017). Joint pain: An update. *Science Insights, 2017*, e00021. doi:10.15354/si.17.re016

124. Landrier, J-F., Tourniaire, F., Fenni, S., Desmarchelier, C., & Borel, P. (2017). Tomatoes and lycopene: Inflammatory modulator effects. Boca Raton, FL: CRC Press.

125. Borch, D., Juul-Hindsgaul, N., Veller, M., Astrup, A., Jaskolowski, J., & Raben, A. Potatoes and risk of obesity, type 2 diabetes, and cardiovascular disease in apparently healthy adults: A systematic review of intervention and observational studies. (2016). *The American Journal of Clinical Nutrition, 104*(2), 489-498. doi:10.3945/ajcn.116.132332

126. USDA FoodData Central. Potatoes, flesh and skin, raw. Retrieved January 2, 2020, from https://fdc.nal.usda.gov/fdc-app.html#/food-details/170026/nutrients

127. Khoo, H.E., Azlan, A., Tang, S.T., & Lim, S.M. (2017). Anthocyanidins and anthocyanins: colored pigments as food, pharmaceutical ingredients, and the potential health benefits. *Food & Nutrition Research, 61*(1), doi:10.1080/16546628.2017.1361779

128. Georgescu, S-R., Sârbu, M-I, Matei, C., Ilie, M.A., Caruntu, C., Constantin, C., Neagu, M., & Tampa, M. (2017). Capsaicin: Friend or foe in skin cancer and other related malignancies? *Nutrients, 9*(12). doi:10.3390/nu912365

129. Kumar, S., Verma, A.K., Das, M., Jain, S.K., & Dwivedi, P.D. (2013). Clinical complications of kidney bean consumption. *Nutrition, 29.* 821-827.

130. Gemede, H.F., & Ratta, N. (2014). Antinutritional factors in plant foods: Potential health benefits and adverse effects. *International Journal of Nutrition and Food Sciences, 3*(4), 284-289. doi:10.11648/j.ijnfs.20140304.18

131. Lal, N., Barcchiya, J., Raypuriya, N., & Shiurkar, G. (2017). Anti-nutrition in legumes: effect in human health and its elimination. *Innovative Farming, 2*(1), 32-36.

132. Suárez-Martínez, S.E., Ferriz-Martínez, R.A., Campos-Vega, R., Elton-Puente, J.E., de la Torre Carbot, K., & García-Gasca, T. (2016). Bean seeds: leading nutraceutical source for human health. *CyTA- Journal of Food, 14*(1), 131-137. doi:10.10080/19476337.2015.1063548

133. Habs, M., Binder, K., Krauss, S., Müller, K., Ernst, B., Valentini, L., & Koller, M. (2017). A balanced risk-benefit analysis to determine human risks associated with pyrrolizidine alkaloids (PA)—The case of tea and herbal infusions. *Nutrients, 9*(7). doi:10.3390/nu9070717

134. Richard, T., Temsamani, H., Cantos-Villar, E., & Monti, J-P. (2013). Chapter two- Application of LC-MS and LC-NMR techniques for secondary metabolite identification. *Advances in Botanical Research, 67,* 67-98. doi:10.1016/B978-0-12-397922-3.00002-2

135. Ruxton, C.H.S. (2008). The impact of caffeine on mood, cognitive function, performance, and hydration: A review of benefits and risks. *Nutrition Bulletin, 33*(1), 15-25. doi:10.1111/j.1467-3010.2007.00665.x

136. Irshad, M., Asgher, M., Bhatti, K.H., Zafar, M., & Anwar, Z. (2017). Anticancer and neutraceutical potentialities of phystase/phytate. *International Journal of Pharmacology, 13*(7), 808-817.

137. van Buul, V.J., & Brouns, F.J.P.H. (2014). Health effects of wheat lectins: A review. *Journal of Cereal Science, 59*(2), 112-117.

138. Smeriglio, A., Barreca, D., Bellocco, E., & Trombetta, D. (2016). Proanthocyadins and hydrolysable tannins: occurrence, dietary intake, and pharmacological effects. *British Journal of Pharmacology, 174*(11), 1244-1262. doi:10.1111/bph.13630

139. Fernandes, A.C., Nishida, W., & Da Costa Proença, R.P. (2010). Influence of soaking on the nutritional quality of common beans (*Phaseolus vulgaris L.*) cooked with or without the soaking water: A review. *Food Science & Technology, 45*(11), 2209-2218. doi:10.1111/j.1365-2621.2010.02395.x

140. Singh, A.K., Rehal, J., Kaur, A., & Jyot, G. (2015). Enhancement of attributes of cereals by germination and fermentation: A review. *Critical Reviews in Food Science and Nutrition. 11,* 1575-1589. doi:10.1080/10408398.2012.706661

141. Haileslassie, H.A., Henry, C.J., & Tyler, R.T. (2016). Impact of household food processing strategies on antinutrient (phytate, tannin, and polyphenol) contents of chickpeas (*Cicer arietinum* L.) and beans (*Phaseolus vulgaris* L.): A review. *Food Science & Technology, 51*(9), 1947-1957. doi:10.1111/ijfs.13166

142. Chai, W., & Liebman, M. (2005). Effect of different cooking methods on vegetable oxalate content. *Journal of Agricultural and Food Chemistry, 53*(8), 3027-3030. doi:10.1021/jf048128d

143. Hamm, L.L., Nakhoul, N., & Hering-Smith, K.S. (2015). Acid-base homeostasis. *Clinical Journal of the American Society of Nephrology, 10*(12), 2232-2242. doi:10.2215/CJN.07400715

144. Schwalfenberg, G.K. (2012). The alkaline diet: Is there evidence that an alkaline pH diet benefits health? *Journal of Environmental and Public Health, 2012*, 727630. doi:10.1155/2012/727630

145. Fenton, T.R., Tough, S.C., Lyon, A.W., Eliasziw, M., & Hanley, D.A. (2011). Causal assessment of dietary acid load and bone disease: A systematic review & meta-analysis applying Hill's epidemiologic criteria for causality. *Nutrition Journal, 10*(41). doi:10.1186/1475-2891-10-41

146. Fenton, T.R., & Huang, T. (2016). Systematic review of the association between dietary acid load, alkaline water, and cancer. *BMJ Open, 6*, e010438. doi:10.1136/bmjopen-2015-010438

147. Passey, C. (2017). Reducing the dietary acid load: How a more alkaline diet benefits patients with chronic kidney disease. *Journal of Renal Nutrition, 27*(3), 151-160. doi:10.1053/j.jrn.2016.11.006

148. Angéloco, L.R.N., Arces de Souza, G.C., Romão, E.A., & Chiarello, P.A. (2018). Alkaline diet and metabolic acidosis: Practical approaches to the nutritional management of chronic kidney disease. *Journal of Renal Nutrition, 28*(3), 215-220. doi:10.1053/j.jrn.2017.10.006

149. Zahara, Y., & Parvin, M. (2018). Alkaline diet: A novel nutritional strategy in chronic kidney disease? *Iranian Journal of Kidney Diseases, 12*(4), 204-208.

150. Kalantar-Zadeh, K., & Moore, L.W. (2019). Does kidney longevity mean healthy vegan food and less meat or is any low-protein diet good enough? *Journal of Renal Nutrition, 29*(2), 79-91. doi:10.1053/j.jrn.2019.01.008

151. Moellering, R.E., Black, K.C., Krishnamurty, C., Baggett, B.K., Stafford, P., Rain, M., . . . Gillies, R.J. (2008). Acid treatment of melanoma cells selects for invasive phenotypes. *Clinical & Experimental Metastasis, 25*(4), 411-425. doi:10.1007/s10585-008-9145-7

152. Martínez-Zaguilán, R., Seftor, E.A., Seftor, R.E., Chu, Y.W., Gillies, R.J., & Hendrix, M.J. (1996). Acidic pH enhances the invasive behavior of human melanoma cells. *Clinical & Experimental Metastasis, 14*(2), 176-186.

153. Magro, M., Corain, L., Ferro, S., Baratella, D., Bonaluto, E., Terzo, M., . . . Vianello, F. (2016). Alkaline water and longevity: A murine study. *Evidence-based Complementary and Alternative Medicine*, 1-6. doi:10.1155/2016/3084126

154. Weidman, J., Holsworth Jr., R.E., Brossman, B., Cho, D., St. Cyr, J., & Fridman, G. (2016). Effect of electrolyzed high-pH alkaline water on blood viscosity in healthy adults. *Journal of the International Society of Sports Nutrition, 13*(45).

155. Yan, H., Kashiwaki, T., Hamasaki, T., Kinjo, T., Teruya, K., Kabayama, S., & Shirahata, S. (2011). The neuroprotective effects of electrolyzed reduced water and its model water containing molecular hydrogen and Pt nanoparticles. *BMC Proceedings, 5*(8), 69. doi:10.1186/1753-6561-5-S8-P69

156. Riaz, B., Ikram, R., & Sikandar, B. (2018). Anticataleptic activity of zamzam water in chlorpromazine induced animal model of Parkinson disease. *Pakistan Journal of Pharmaceutical Sciences, 31*(2), 393-397.

157. Wang, Y. (2001). Preliminary observation on changes of blood pressure, blood sugar, and blood lipids after using alkaline ionized drinking water. *Shanghai Journal of Preventative Medicine,* 2001(12).

158. Jin, D., Ryu, S.H., Kim, H.W., Yang, E.J., Lim, S.J., Ryang, Y.S., Chung, C.H., Psark, S.K., & Lee, K.J. (2006). Anti-diabetic effect of alkaline-reduced water on OLETF rats. *Bioscience, Biotechnology, and Biochemistry, 70*(1), 31-37.

159. Koufman, J.A., & Johnston, N. (2012). Potential benefits of pH 8.8 alkaline drinking water as an adjunct in the treatment of reflux disease. *Annals of Otology, Rhinology, & Laryngology, 121*(7), 431-434. doi:10.1177/000348941212100702

160. Verheggen, R.J.H.M., Maessen, M.F.H., Green, D.J., Hermus, A.R.M.M., Hopman, M.T.E., & Thijssen, D.H.T. (2016). A systematic review and meta-analysis on the effects of exercise training versus hypocaloric diet: distinct effects on body weight and visceral adipose tissue. *Obesity Reviews, 17*(8), 664-690.

161. Wewege, M., van den Berg, R., Ward, R.E., & Keech, A. (2017). The effects of high-intensity interval training vs. moderate-intensity continuous training on body composition in overweight and obese adults: a systematic review and meta-analysis. *Obesity Reviews, 18*(6), 635-646. doi:10.1111/obr.12532

162. Viana, R., Naves, J.P., Coswig, V., & de Lira, C.A.B. (2019). Is interval training the magic bullet for fat loss? A systematic review and meta-analysis comparing moderate-intensity continuous training with high-intensity interval training (HIIT). *British Journal of Sports Medicine, 53*(10). doi:10.1136/bjsports-2018-099928

163. Said, M.A., Abdelmoneem, M., Almaqhawi, A., Kotob, A.A.H., Alibrahim, M.C., & Bougmiza, I. (2018). Multidisciplinary approach to obesity: Aerobic or resistance physical exercise? *Journal of Exercise Science & Fitness, 16*(3), 118-123.

164. Willis, L.H., Slentz, C.A., Bateman, L.A., Shields, T.S., Piner, L.W., Bales, C.W., . . . Kraus, W.E. (2012). Effects of aerobic and/or resistance training on body mass and fat mass in overweight or obese adults. *Journal of Applied Physiology, 113*(12), 1831-1837. doi:10.1152/japplphysiol.01370.2011

165. Ismael, I., Keating, S.E., Baker, M.K., & Johnson, M.A. (2012). A systematic review and meta-analysis of the effect of aerobic vs. resistance exercise training on visceral fat. *Obesity Reviews, 13*(1), 68-91. doi:10.1111/j.1467-789X.2011.00931.x

166. Shuster, A., Patlas, M., Pinthus, J.H., & Mourtzakis, M. (2012). The clinical importance of visceral adiposity: A critical review of methods for visceral adipose tissue analysis. *British Journal of Radiology, 85*(1009), 1-10. doi:10.1259/bjr/38447238

167. Villareal, D.T., Aguirre, L., Gurney, A.B., Waters, D.L., Sinacore, D.R., Colombo, E., . . . Qualls, C. (2017). Aerobic or resistance exercise, or both, in dieting obese older adults. *New England Journal of Medicine, 376,* 1943-1955. doi:10.1056/NEJMoa1616338

168. Institute of Medicine (US) Subcommittee on Military Weight Management. (2004). *Weight management: State of the Science and Opportunities for Military Programs.* Washington, DC: National Academics Press.

169. Balaskas, P., & Jackson, M.E. (2018). Genetics and epigenetics in the aetiology of obesity. In John Wiley & Sons, Ltd. (Eds.), *Advanced Nutrition and Dietetics in Obesity,* 87-95.

170. Rao, K.R., Lal, N., & Giridharan, N.V. (2014). Genetic & epigenetic approach to human obesity. *The Indian Journal of Medical Research, 140*(5), 589-603.

171. Willer, C.J., Speliotes, E.K., Loos, R., . . . & Hirschhorn, J.N. (2009). Six new loci associated with body mass index highlight a neuronal influence on body weight regulation. *Nature Genetics, 41*(1), 25-34. doi:10.1038/ng.287

172. Haupt, A., Thamer, C., Staiger, H., Tschritter, O., Kirchhoff, K., Machicao, F., Häring, H.U., Stefan, N., & Fritsche, A. (2009). Variation in the FTO gene influences food intake but not energy expenditure. *Experimental and Clinical Endocrinology & Diabetes, 117*(4), 194-197. doi:10.1055/s-0028-1087176

173. Leeners, B., Geary, N., Tobler, P.N., & Asarian, L. (2017). Ovarian hormones and obesity. *Human Reproduction Update, 23*(3), 300-321. doi:10.1093/humupd/dmw045

174. Karvonen-Gutierrez, C., & Kim, C. (2016). Association of mid-life changes in body size, body composition, and obesity status with the menopausal transition. *Healthcare, 4*(3), 42. doi:10.3390/healthcare4030042

175. Kapoor, E., Collazo-Clavell, M.L., & Faubion, S.S. (2017). Weight gain in women at midlife: A concise review of the pathophysiology and strategies for management. *Mayo Clinic Proceedings, 92*(10), 1552-1558. doi:10.1016/j.mayocp.2017.08.004

176. Lee, J., Han, Y., Cho, H.H., & Kim, M. (2019). Sleep disorders and menopause. *Journal of Menopausal Medicine, 25*(2), 83-87. doi:10.6118/jmm.19192

177. Prinz, P. (2004). Sleep, appetite, and obesity—What's the link? *PLoS Medicine, 1*(3), e61.

178. de Villiers, T.J., Hall, J.E., Pinkerton, J.V., Cerdas Pérez, S., Rees, M., Yang, C., & Pierroz, D.D. (2016). Revised global consensus statement on menopausal hormone therapy. *Climacteric. 19*(4), 313-315., 153-155. doi:10.1080/13697137.2016.1196047

179. Li, S., Zhao, J.H., Luan, J., Ekelund, U., Luben, R.N., Khaw, K.T., Wareham, N.J., & Loos, R.J.F. (2010). Physical activity attenuates the genetic predisposition to obesity in 20,000 men and women from EPIC-Norfolk prospective population study. *PLoS Medicine, 7*(8), e1000332.

180. West, N., Dorling, J., Thackray, A.E., Hanson, N.C., Decombel, S.E., Stensel, D.J., & Grice, S.J. (2018). Effect of obesity-linked FTO rs9939609 variant on physical activity and dietary patterns in physically active men and women. *Journal of Obesity, 2018* doi:10.1155/2018/7560707

181. McQueen, M.A. (2009). Exercise aspects of obesity treatment. *The Ochsner Journal, 9*(3), 140-143.

182. Bray, G.A., Frühbeck, G., Ryan, D.H., & Wilding, J.P.H. (2016). Management of obesity. *The Lancet, 387*(10031), 1947-1956. doi:10.1016/S0140-6736(16)00271-3

183. Westwater, M.L., Fletcher, P.C., & Ziauddeen, H. (2016). Sugar addiction: The state of the science. *European Journal of Nutrition, 55*(Suppl. 2), 55-69.

184. Dinicolantonio, J., O'Keefe, J., & Wilson, W. (2017). Sugar addition: Is it real? A narrative review. *British Journal of Sports Medicine, 52*(14). doi:10.1136/bjsports-2017-097971

185. Murphy, M.H., Lahart, I., Carlin, I., & Murtagh, E. (2019). The effects of continuous compared to accumulated exercise on health: A meta-analytic review. *Sports Medicine, 49*(10), 1585-1607. doi:10.1007/s40279-019-01145-2

186. Müller, M.J., Geisler, C., Heymsfield, S.B., & Bosy-Westphal, A. (2018). Recent advances in understanding body weight homeostasis in humans. *F1000Research, 7*(F100). doi:10.12688/f1000research.14151.1

187. Speakman, J.R., Levitsky, D.A., Allison, D.B., Bray, M.S., de Castro, J.M., Clegg, D.J., . . . Westerterp-Plantenga, M.S. (2011). Set points, settling points, and some alternative models: Theoretical options to understand how genes and environments combine to regulate body adiposity. *Disease Models & Mechanisms, 4*(6), 733-745. doi:10.1242/dmm.008698

188. Mansoubi, M., Pearson, N., Clemes, S.A., Biddle, S.J., Bodicoat, D.H., Tolfrey, K., . . . Yates, T. (2015). Energy expenditure during common sitting and standing tasks: examining the 1.5 MET definition of sedentary behavior. *BMC Public Health, 15*, 516. doi:10.1186/s12889-015-1851-x

189. Sarker, M., & Rahman, M. (2017). Dietary fiber and obesity management- A review. *MedCrave, 7*(3).

190. Stahl, B.A., Peco, E., Davla, S., Murakami, K., Caicedo Moreno, N.A., van Meyel, D.J., & Keene, A.C. (2018). Sleep and metabolism: Eaat-ing your way to ZZZs. *Current Biology, 22*(19), R1310-R1312. doi:10.1016/j.cub.2018.08.030

191. Tomiyama, A.J. (2018). Stress and obesity. *Annual Review of Psychology, 70*(5), 703-718. doi:10.1146/annurev-psych-010418-102936

192. American Psychiatric Association. (2013). *Diagnostic and statistical manual of mental disorders* (5th ed.). Washington, DC.

193. McCorry, L.K. (2007). Physiology of the autonomic nervous system. *American Journal of Pharmaceutical Education, 71*(4), 78. doi:10.5688/aj710478

194. Volkow, N.D., Wang, G.J., & Baler, R.D. (2011). Reward, dopamine, and the control of food intake: Implications for obesity. *Trends in Cognitive Sciences, 15*(1), 37-46.

195. Rosenbaum, M., Sy, M., Paclovich, K., Leibel, R.L., & Hirsch, J. (2008). Leptin reverses weight loss-induced changes in regional neural activity responses to visual stimuli. *The Journal of Clinical Investigation, 118*(7), 2583-2591. doi:10.1172/JCI35055

196. Myers, M.G., Cowley, M.A., & Münzberg, H. (2008). Mechanisms of leptin action and leptin resistance. *Annual Review of Physiology, 70*, 537-556. doi:10.1146/annurev.physiol.70.113006.100707

197. Adam, T.C., & Epel, E.S. (2007). Stress, eating and the reward system. *Psychology & Behavior, 91*, 449-458.

198. Hildebrandt, B.A., Racine, S.E., Burt, A., Neale, M., Boker, S., Sisk, C.L. & Klump, K.L. (2015). The effects of ovarian hormones and emotional eating on changes in weight preoccupation across the menstrual cycle. *The International Journal of Eating Disorders, 48*(5), 477-487. doi:10.1002/eat.22326

199. Ashcroft, J., Semmler, C., Carnell, S., & van Jaarsveld, C.H.M. (2007). Continuity and stability of eating behavior traits in children. *European Journal of Clinical Nutrition, 62*, 985-990.

200. Bellisle, F. (2009). Assessing various aspects of the motivation to eat that can affect food intake and body weight control. *L Encéphale, 35*(2), 182-185. doi:10.1016/j.encep.2008.03.009

201. Carnell, S., Haworth, C.M.A., & Wardle, J. (2008). Genetic influence on appetite in children. *International Journal of Obesity, 32*, 1468-1473. doi:10.1038/ijo.2008.127

202. Grimm, E.R., & Steinle, N.I. (2011). Genetics of eating behavior: Established and emerging concepts. *Nutrition Reviews, 69*(1), 52-60. doi:10.1111/j.1753-4887.2010.00361.x

203. Van Strein, T. (2018). Causes of emotional eating and matched treatment of obesity. *Obesity, 1.* doi:10.1007/s11892-018-1000-x

204. Höppener, M.M., Larsen, J.K., van Strien, T., Ouwens, M.A., Winkens, L.H.H., & Disinga, R. (2019). Depressive symptons and emotional eating: Mediated by mindfulness? *Mindfulness, 10*(4), 670-678. doi:10.1007/s12671-018-1002-4

205. Goldbacher, E., La Grotte, C., Komaroff, E., Vander Veur, S., & Foster, G.D. (2015). An initial evaluation of a weight loss intervention for individuals who engage in emotional eating. *Journal of Behavioral Medicine, 39*, 139-150. doi:10.1007/s10865-015-9678-6

206. Scott, K.A., Melhorn, S.J., & Sakai, R.R. (2012). Effects of chronic social stress on obesity. *Current Obesity Reports, 1*(1), 16-25. doi:10.1007/s13679-011-0006-3

207. Paolucci, E.M., Loukov, D., Bowdish, D.M.E., & Heisz, J.J. (2018). Exercise reduces depression and inflammation but intensity matters. Biological Psychology, 133, 79-84. doi:10.1016/j.biopsycho.2018.01.015

208. Leach, C.W. (2017). Understanding shame and guilt. In L. Woodyatt, E. Worthington Jr., M. Wenzel, & B. Griffin (Eds.), *Handbook of the psychology of self-forgiveness.* Springer, Cham. doi:10.1007/978-3-319-60573-9_2

209. Schoenfeld, B. (2011). Does cardio after an overnight fast maximize fat loss? *Strength and Conditioning Journal, 33*(1), 23-25. doi:10.1519/SSC.0b013e31820396ec

INDEX

Note: The italicized *t* following page numbers refers to tables.

ABOUT THE AUTHORS

Melody Schoenfeld, MA, CSCS, is a certified personal trainer with over 25 years of training experience in many different disciplines. She holds a master's degree in health psychology and writes and speaks both nationally and internationally on a wide variety of health and fitness subjects. She is the owner of Flawless Fitness, a personal training center in Pasadena, California. In 2019, she was recognized as NSCA's Personal Trainer of the Year.

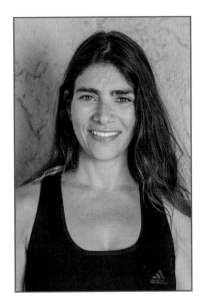

Schoenfeld has held state and national records in all three lifts in powerlifting (squat, bench press, and deadlift) and competes in powerlifting and strongman competitions. An aficionado of old-time strongman shows of strength, she performs feats such as tearing phone books and license plates in half and bending steel rebar, horseshoes, and nails. She is the self-published author of *Pleasure Not Meating You.* In her free time, you'll find her cooking unreasonably large quantities of vegan food, fronting a few heavy metal bands, and telling horrible jokes.

Susan Kleiner, PhD, RD, CNS, FACN, FISSN, is the founder and owner of the internationally recognized consulting firm High Performance Nutrition LLC. A visionary educator and motivator, she speaks nationally and internationally on topics in the field of nutrition, health, and performance. She is a sought-after expert interview as well as writer in all forms of print, online, and broadcast media. She has authored eight books, including the bestseller The New Power Eating, The Good Mood Diet, and The PowerFood Nutrition Plan.

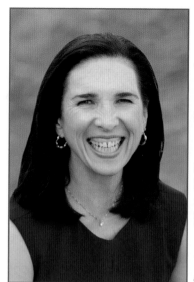

Courtesy of Katie M. Simmons Photography.

Kleiner has been the high-performance nutrition consultant to professional athletes and teams nationally and internationally, including the Seattle Storm, Seattle Reign, Seattle Seahawks, Seattle Mariners, Seattle Supersonics, Cleveland Browns, Cleveland Cavaliers, Miami Heat, Olympians, and elite and recreational athletes of all ages in countless sports.

She is a cofounder and fellow of the International Society of Sports Nutrition and a fellow of the American College of Nutrition. She is also a member of the American College of Sports Medicine and the National Strength and Conditioning Association.

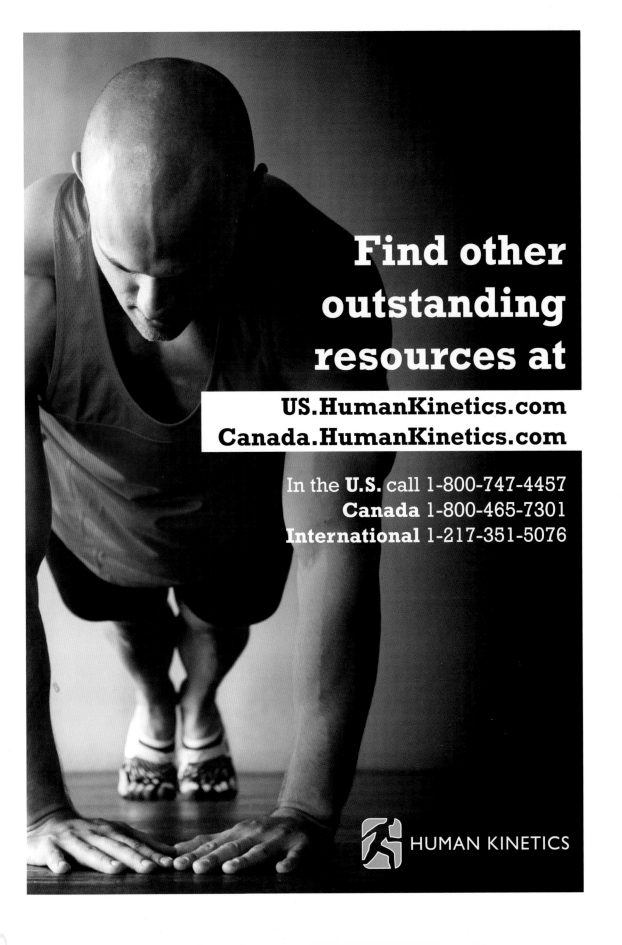

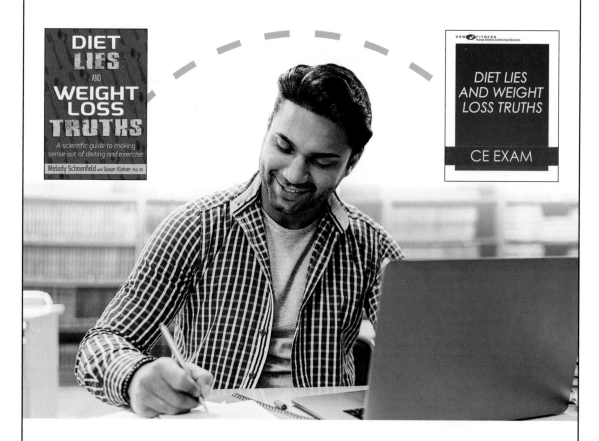
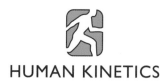